i

THE LIGHT WITHIN – A VEDIC MAP TO HAPPINESS

First Edition, 2025
ISBN 978-1-7342115-8-0

For any further information, contact: www.wellbeen.com

ACKNOWLEDGEMENTS

To Mother Earth, the eternal source of nourishment and healing.

To my Guru, Bhagawan Sri Sathya Sai Baba, whose divine presence illumines my path.

To Sadguru Sri Madhusudan Sai, with deep love and gratitude, for his constant encouragement, his call to serve others, and his vision that inspires me to honor nature's wisdom in the journey of healing.

To my father, whose unwavering guidance strengthens me.

To my loving and kind family, for always encouraging me, for embracing the natural ways of nourishment, and for patiently being pulled into countless botanical and herbal gardens along the way.

And above all, to the innate intelligence of the Universe, for gifting humanity with plants, herbs, and superfoods—sacred companions in our well-being.

For me, gratitude is not merely an attitude, but the very rhythm and truth of the Universe.

PREFACE

"We are all, in some way, seekers of happiness.

Though its meaning may differ for each of us, in its essence, happiness is contentment, joy, or bliss — a sense of inner fulfillment.

Most of our actions, whether small or great, are ultimately driven by the desire to experience this state of happiness.

We all wander, seeking happiness,
Each heart defining it in its own hue.
For some, a fleeting smile of contentment,
For others, the boundless joy of being true.

Yet in its essence, it is one —
The stillness where the soul feels whole,
A quiet bliss, a tranquil sun,
That shines within the seeker's soul.

All our actions, dreams, and desires,
Are but ripples from that yearning deep —
To touch that light, that never tires,
The happiness we all seek to keep."

This book is born out of my journey across all levels of existence — physical, emotional, mental, intellectual, and spiritual.

The divine guidance for this path came from Bhagawan Sri Sathya Sai Baba, who gently nudged me toward pursuing a Ph.D. in Metaphysics, though my formal training was in Botany.

Following that divine prompting, I ventured into territories far beyond the scientific boundaries I once knew — exploring Vedantic concepts, alternative healing, and the subtle realms where consciousness itself becomes medicine. What began as a quest for good health gradually unfolded into a revelation — an entire universe of possibilities within.

My research led me to the Bhruguvalli and the profound wisdom of the Anadavalli, where I began to perceive food, life, and consciousness as one sacred continuum. Initially, my pursuit was only to heal my body, but this exploration opened a luminous path toward understanding the true nature of happiness, Ānanda, and bliss.

These energies became my closest companions — my "energy friends." I began seeking them in every thought, every action, every breath. Slowly, I realized that happiness is not something we chase outside ourselves — it blossoms only when the mind turns inward and aligns with its own source.

This book encapsulates over thirty years of deep research, reflection, and experimentation. It is not merely a study, but a living experience of inner transformation.

Through this journey, I have come to understand a simple truth — no one else can create your bliss for you. Each of us must learn to dwell in that state consciously. When we align with our own inner Ananda, Moksha is not a distant goal; it becomes a living experience — here and now, in the sacred gift of the present moment. My journey through countless healing paths became the mirror through which I discovered this truth.

I explored Reiki, Yoga, Channeling, Sai Vibronics, Homeopathy, Naturopathy, Traditional and Occult Healing, Mantras, Divination, Astrology, Access Consciousness, Theta Healing, and more. Each modality guided me closer to my own center — to the still point within where all healing truly begins.
I experimented with Aromatherapy, Zen meditation, Crystals and Gem Therapy, Vāstu and Feng Shui — every ancient and modern art that resonated with the vibration of

harmony. Each one added a note of wisdom, refining my understanding that healing is not about adding more, but about returning to the state of inner balance and joy.

As I slowed down, focus deepened — and the intensity of awareness became so alive that miracles began to unfold naturally. They were not the result of techniques, but the outcome of alignment — when the outer world starts mirroring your inner serenity.

So, I now know:

It is only when you dwell in your own Ānanda — your bliss-consciousness — that true transformation can flow through you. Only from that space does healing become effortless, natural, and divine.

— Rev. Dr. Gauri M. Relan

CONTENTS

INTRODUCTION

All spiritual traditions point toward: that the desire to "help" can sometimes arise from ego, not pure compassion. It shows awareness of how easily energy dynamics can become entangled when we identify as the giver or rescuer.

This book is not a manual of theories — it is a living guide to help you rediscover your own inner healing intelligence. Each page is designed to awaken awareness at the five levels of existence — physical, emotional, mental, intellectual, and spiritual — so that healing becomes a state of being, not merely a process.

You will find reflections, practices, and insights drawn from Vedic wisdom, metaphysical research, and nature's healing intelligence. These are the same tools that helped me align my body and mind to the rhythm of the soul.

At the physical level, this book helps you understand how your body communicates through sensations, cravings, and ailments — showing the path of listening, not controlling.

At the emotional level, it teaches you how feelings are sacred messengers, guiding you toward harmony.

At the mental level, it offers clarity on the nature of thoughts — how to transform anxiety into awareness and confusion into calm.

At the intellectual level, it reawakens discernment — the buddhi that helps you see life as it is.

And at the spiritual level, it reminds you that you are not separate from the Source — that bliss (Ānanda) is your true essence, ever-present beneath the noise of the mind.

This is not about adopting another belief system, but about experiencing your own truth. When you begin to live in alignment — when your thoughts, emotions, and actions vibrate in unison — you enter a state of deep, sustained joy.

You do not need to wait for the perfect time, place, or teacher. You already carry the light of wisdom within you. All you need is to remember.

This book will gently guide you to that remembrance —
to a space where healing is natural, where happiness is effortless, and where every moment becomes a doorway to Moksha — liberation here and now.

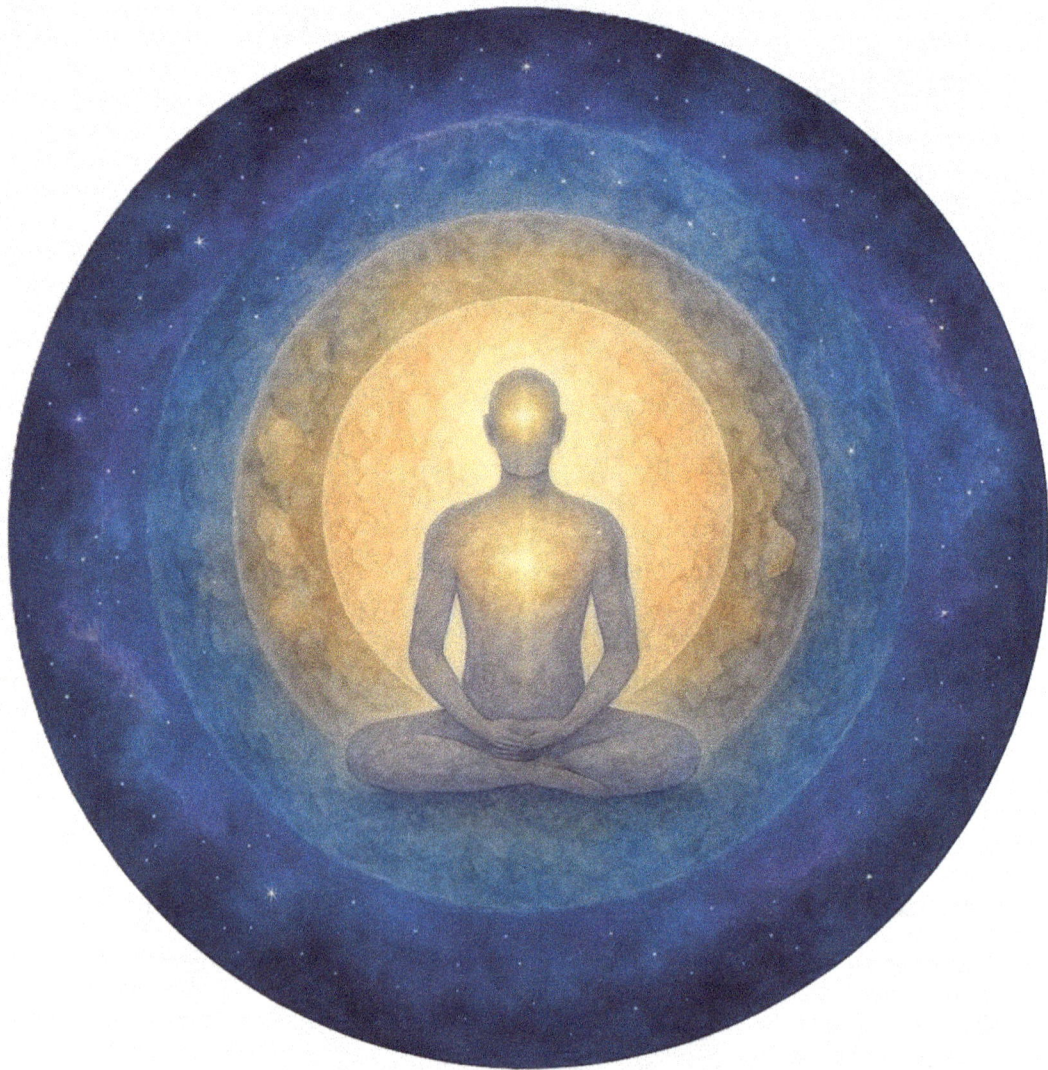

BE IN YOUR BLISS

People often create drama to draw upon your energy. Remember — when you begin to multiply your prana (your inner radiance, life force, or strength), new energies naturally enter your life. Along with them, the ego softly whispers: "I can help. I can heal. I can change others." Yet this, too, is the ego — seeking to feel special through helping.

True service does not arise from lack, but from fullness — from the state of blissful joy. When you are anchored in that joy, your very presence becomes healing. No effort is required. No one is truly a "somebody," for life itself helps everyone, and life itself dissolves everyone.

So, stay centered in joy. Allow others to walk their own paths. Do not fall into the illusion of saving anyone — simply radiate your state of being.

For me — or rather, for all of us — helping is not a desire; it is our nature. It flows effortlessly, like the fragrance of a flower, when we are rooted in contentment and joy — the bliss state. Perhaps we are all born for this: to serve as expressions of the Joy of Life that moves through us.

THE HARMONY OF LIFE'S PATH AND PURPOSE

The Vedas do not see life as divided — but as a single sacred rhythm. The Āśramas are the seasons of life, and the Purushārthas are the fruits of those seasons.

Each stage refines our understanding of happiness — from innocence to insight, from desire to detachment, until joy is no longer dependent on outer things, but springs from the Self itself.

MIRACLES OF ALIGNMENT: THE POWER OF ĀNANDA

When the mind settles and the heart opens, an invisible alignment begins. It is not the alignment of the planets or the people around you — it is the alignment of you with your own Ānanda, your eternal bliss-consciousness.

Ānanda is not a fleeting joy born from success or comfort. It is the steady pulse of existence itself — the quiet radiance that grounds you in truth, the vibration that connects you directly to the Source. When you are in this state, you become a powerhouse of pure energy, effortlessly magnetic. Everything you truly need begins to gravitate toward you.

Opportunities, people, synchronicities, and even healing — they come not because you chase them, but because your inner frequency calls them home. Just as flowers attract bees without trying, your bliss becomes the fragrance that draws all that is meant for you.

This is the power of being genuinely happy — not the surface-level happiness that depends on circumstances, but the deeper joy that arises when you are simply present, content, and whole.

True happiness is the highest vibration in creation. It is both the path and the destination, the cause and the effect. When you dwell in this inner contentment, you cease to struggle or compare. The mind stops grasping, the heart expands, and your energy begins to circulate like sunlight — nourishing everything it touches. In that state, even silence becomes communication, presence becomes prayer, and your life itself becomes a healing field.

Ānanda grounds you. It roots you in the power of now — unshaken, luminous, and deeply alive. From that grounding, you no longer need to do miracles; you simply become one.

SAT–CHIT–ĀNANDA (BEING–CONSCIOUSNESS–BLISS)

The Eternal Quest for Ānanda

All beings move, in subtle streams,
Seeking happiness through countless dreams.
Each heart defines it in its way,
Yet all return to the same ray.

For in the depths where silence sings,
Dwells the joy no pleasure brings.
Not born of sense, nor mind's delight,
But of the Self — pure, vast, and bright.

Sat — the truth our hearts recall,
Chit — the light that knows it all,
Ānanda — bliss that needs no name,
The flame within, the cosmic flame.

All actions rise, all desires unfold,
From that one thirst, ancient and bold —
To rest in peace, to simply be,
In the boundless Self — eternally free.

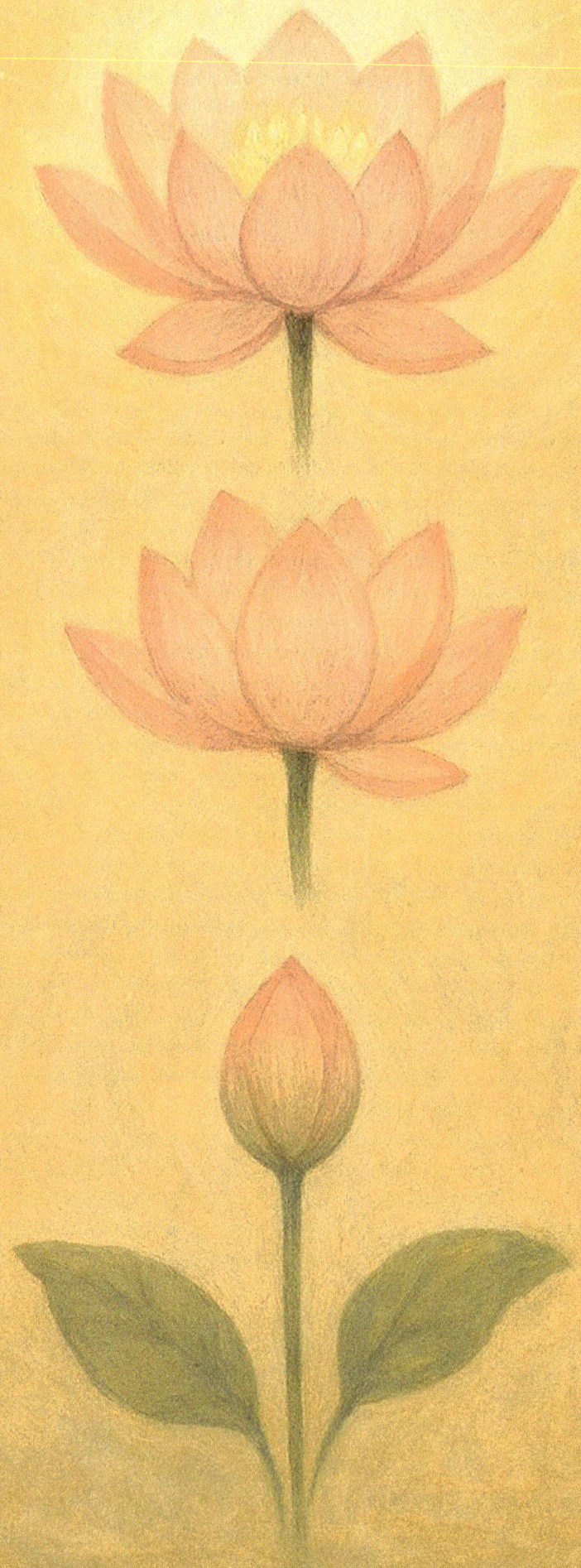

THE CYCLE OF LIFE

THE CHANGING FACES OF HAPPINESS DURING THE CYCLE OF LIFE

Happiness wears many forms, and changes with the rhythm of our years.

As children, it gleams in simple toys, in laughter spilled across the floor, and in the gentle cradle of our mother's lap — our first universe of warmth and safety. As teenagers, happiness dances in friendship, in shared secrets and fleeting dreams, while we storm through emotions, testing the patience of those who love us most. As young adults, our choices unfold, we seek meaning, passion, and place — chasing stars outside, while the true light quietly waits within. For in every stage, joy shifts its guise, teaching us — that happiness is not found, but revealed, as we grow closer to our own Self divine.

So, the Vedic vision of happiness evolves from innocence → engagement → reflection → realization. Each ashram refines our understanding of joy — until we discover that happiness is not outside, but the Ānanda Swarūpa — our very essence.

THE CIRCLE OF LIFE AND LIBERATION

Life begins with curiosity (Brahmacharya), flowers into creativity (Gṛhastha), matures into contemplation (Vānaprastha), and culminates in liberation (Sannyāsa). Throughout this sacred journey, happiness changes its form — from outer pleasure to inner peace, from doing to being, from seeking to shining.

When Dharma guides every stage, when Artha and Kāma serve, not enslave, and when Moksha illuminates all, life itself becomes Yajña — a sacred offering of bliss to the Divine.

THE FOUR ĀŚRAMAS — THE SACRED JOURNEY OF LIFE AND HAPPINESS

1. BRAHMACHARYA – THE JOY OF LEARNING (STUDENT LIFE)

In this dawn of life, the soul is curious. Happiness blooms through learning, discipline, and wonder. Like the rising sun, the mind awakens — seeking truth in the guidance of a Guru. Desires are simple, pure, and the joy lies in discovery.

2. GṚHASTHA – THE JOY OF CREATION (HOUSEHOLDER LIFE)

This is the noon of life, radiant and full. Happiness now wears many forms — family, love, service, and abundance. The world becomes a sacred playground of karma. Here, dharma (duty) and artha (prosperity) balance with kāma (desire), as the soul learns to give and nurture.

3. VĀNAPRASTHA – THE JOY OF WITHDRAWAL (RETIREMENT INTO NATURE)

As the evening descends, the inner call grows stronger. The heart begins to seek peace in silence, turning from outer pleasures to inner reflection. Happiness is now found in solitude, forests, prayers, and contemplation — the soul preparing for its homeward journey.

4. SANNYĀSA – THE JOY OF LIBERATION (RENUNCIATION)

This is the night of deep awareness, where the self dissolves into the Self. Having tasted the world, the seeker now seeks only truth. Detached from name, form, and desire, one rests in Sat-Chit-Ānanda — Being, Consciousness, Bliss. This is the highest happiness — eternal and unchanging.

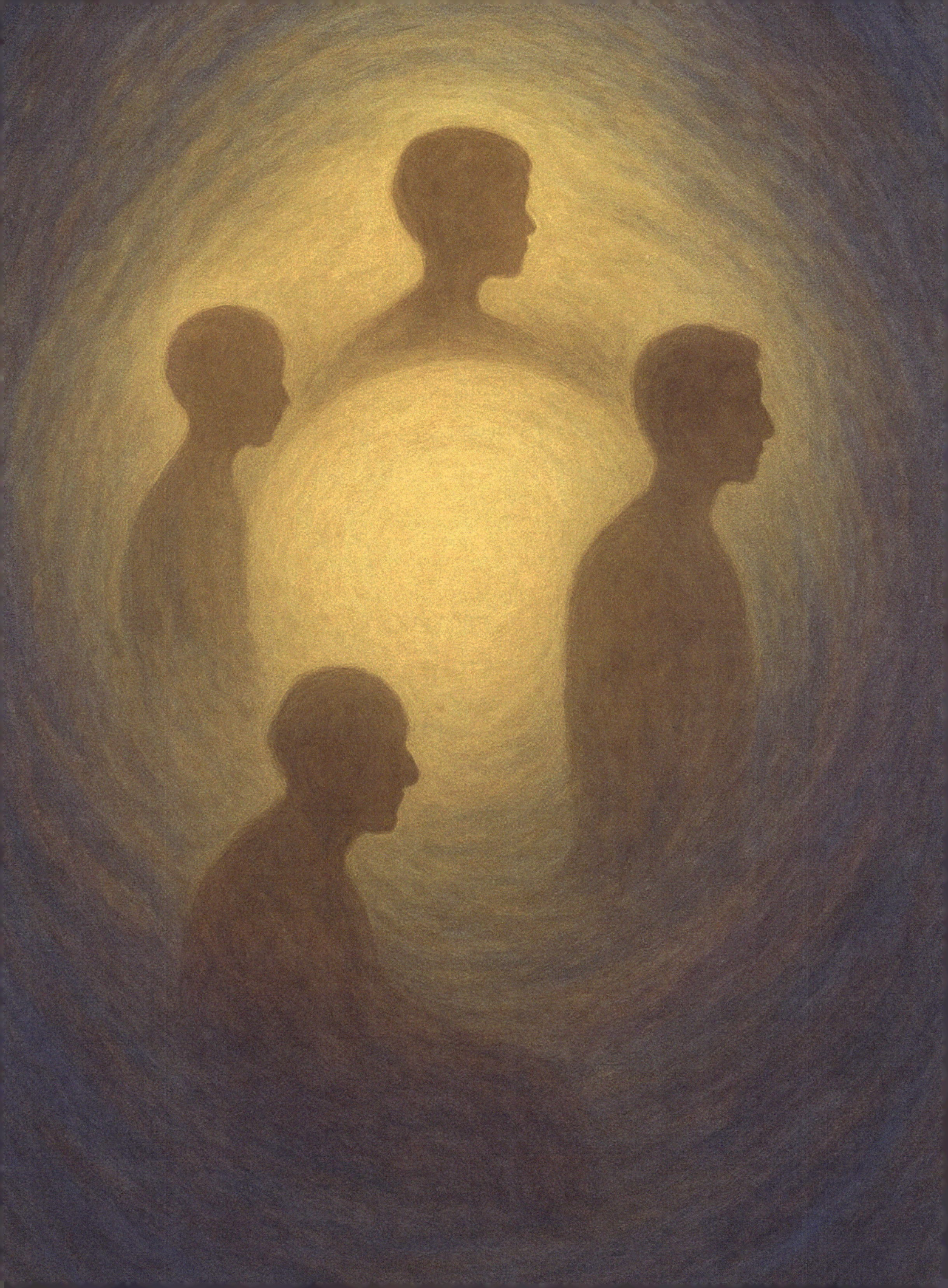

LIFE STAGES

The Four Āśramas (life stages) described in the Vedic tradition form a sacred map for evolving from worldly involvement to spiritual liberation — from karma to moksha, from doing to being.

Each āśrama offers experiences and disciplines that refine the layers of our being (the koshas) and gradually lead us toward Ānanda — bliss, the realization of our true Self.

Let's explore this sacred journey step by step.

1. BRAHMACHARYA — THE STUDENT STAGE (PATH OF LEARNING AND DISCIPLINE)

Focus: Education, self-control, purity, and foundation of Dharma.

Kosha evolved: Manomaya & Vijñānamaya — the mind and intellect.
- This stage teaches restraint, humility, focus, and devotion to learning.
- The senses are trained, the mind purified, and the intellect sharpened through study of the Vedas and inner reflection.
- When the restless mind is disciplined, clarity and peace begin to dawn.

Path to Bliss: *"Self-mastery is the seed of freedom."*
Through purity and focused learning, one attains inner harmony — the first taste of joy born from discipline.

2. GṚHASTHA — THE HOUSEHOLDER STAGE (PATH OF RESPONSIBILITY AND LOVE)

Focus: Family, work, service, and righteous enjoyment (Kama & Artha within Dharma).

Kosha evolved: Annamaya & Prāṇamaya — body and life-force through right action.

- In this stage, one learns to live Dharma in the world — through love, generosity, and service.
- It is the field where lessons of detachment, compassion, and balance are lived in real life.

Path to Bliss: *"When service becomes worship, the world becomes sacred."*

By performing duties with love and detachment, life itself becomes yoga — a path to divine joy.

3. VĀNAPRASTHA — THE HERMIT STAGE (PATH OF WITHDRAWAL AND CONTEMPLATION)

Focus: Simplicity, introspection, detachment from possessions and roles.

Kosha evolved: Vijñānamaya — wisdom and discrimination deepen.

- One withdraws from active worldly duties, devoting more time to study, nature, meditation, and silence.
- The mind turns inward, and wisdom ripens through reflection and solitude.

Path to Bliss: *"Silence is the language of the soul."*

By renouncing restlessness and seeking truth, one experiences serenity — a stable joy that arises from understanding.

4. SANNYĀSA — THE RENUNCIATE STAGE (PATH OF LIBERATION AND UNION)

Focus: Total surrender, renunciation of ego, realization of the Self.

Kosha evolved: Ānandamaya — the bliss sheath, pure being.
- The individual sees the Self in all beings and all beings in the Self.
- Nothing to gain, nothing to lose — only Sat-Chit-Ānanda remains.

Path to Bliss: *"I am That — eternal, pure, and free."*

In renouncing the illusion of separateness, the sage abides in bliss — not as emotion, but as being itself.

Āśrama	Focus	Transformation	Bliss Experience
Brahmacharya	Learning & Discipline	Mastery of mind	Joy of clarity
Gṛhastha	Responsibility & Love	Balance in action	Joy of service
Vānaprastha	Detachment & Contemplation	Wisdom dawns	Joy of silence
Sannyāsa	Renunciation & Realization	Union with Self	Infinite Bliss

IN ESSENCE

Through Dharma, one finds order;

through Artha and Kama, one learns balance;

through renunciation, one discovers truth;

and in truth — bliss.

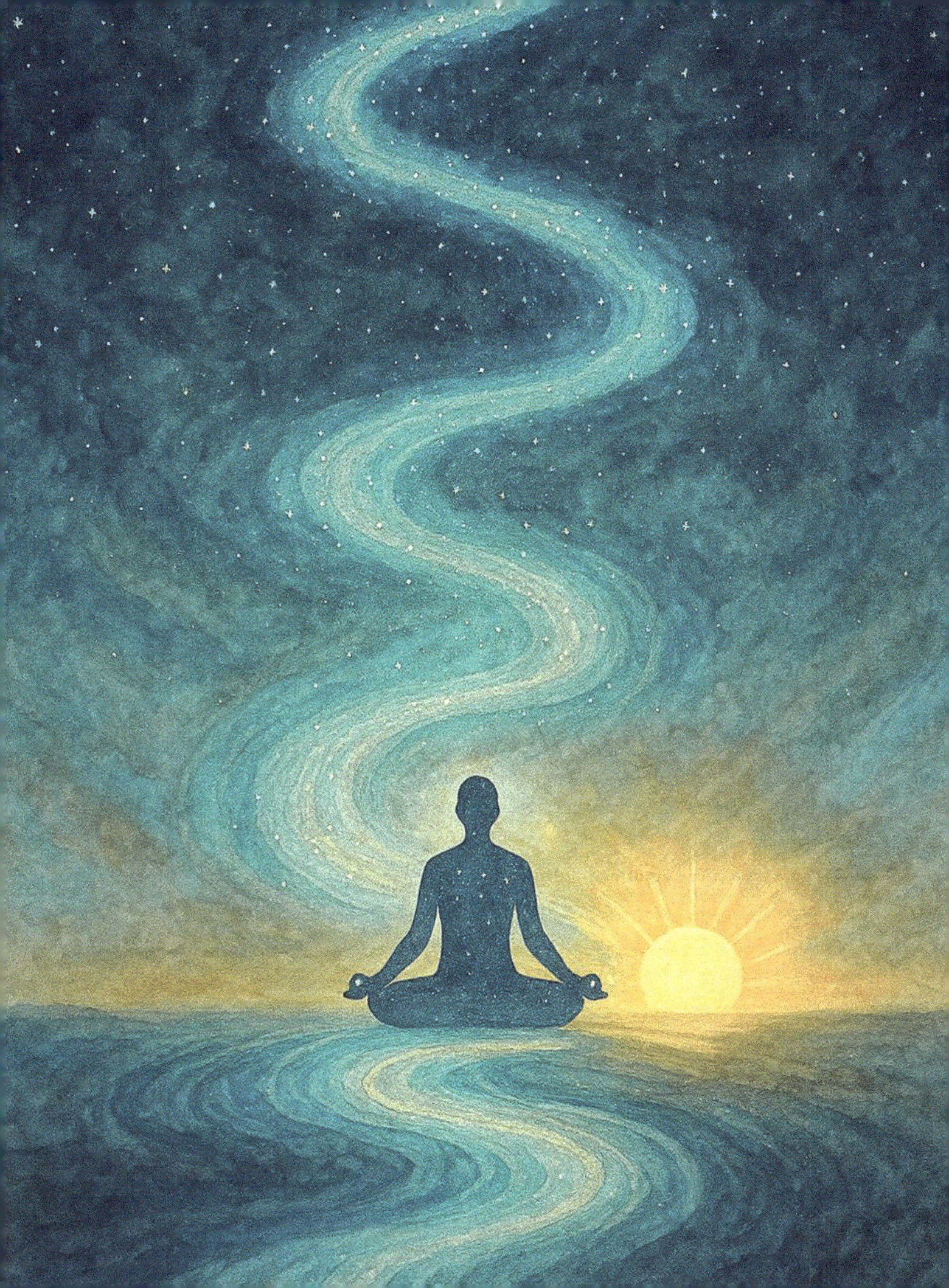

PURUSHARTHA

Purushartha is a profound concept in Vedic philosophy that describes the four goals of human life — the guiding pillars that help us live with meaning, balance, and fulfillment. The Sanskrit word Purushartha means "the purpose or aim (artha) of human life (purusha)."

THE FOUR PURUSHARTHAS

1. Dharma (Righteous living / Moral duty)

Dharma represents living in alignment with truth, virtue, and universal order. It means acting in a way that uplifts not only oneself but also society and nature. Joy arises from inner harmony — when your thoughts, words, and actions reflect integrity.

2. Artha (Prosperity / Material well-being)

Artha is about earning wealth and creating security through honest means. It ensures stability and supports the other goals of life — family, service, and self-growth. Joy here comes from the feeling of self-sufficiency and being able to give and share.

3. Kama (Pleasure / Emotional fulfillment)

Kama encompasses love, beauty, art, relationships, and all forms of sensory joy that elevate the spirit — when pursued mindfully, not indulgently. True joy in Kama is about savoring life with gratitude, without attachment.

4. Moksha (Liberation / Spiritual freedom)

Moksha is the highest goal — freedom from inner bondage, ego, and ignorance. It is the realization that the self is divine, complete, and eternal. This is the joy of pure being — peace that surpasses all external pleasure.

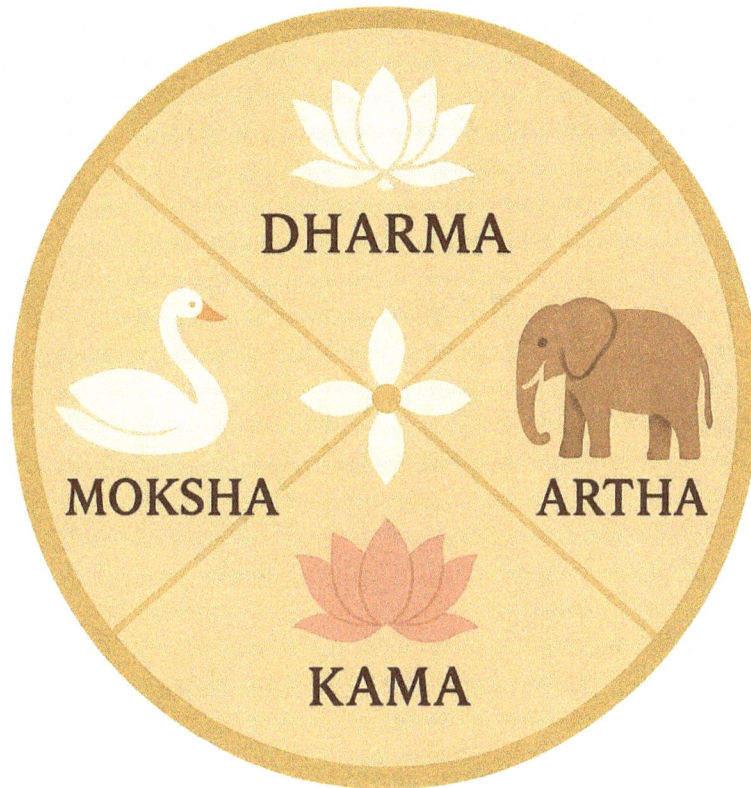

HOW PURUSHARTHA LEADS TO HAPPINESS AND JOY

When all four Purusharthas are balanced, a person experiences holistic well-being — material, emotional, moral, and spiritual.

- Without Dharma, wealth or pleasure can become destructive.
- Without Artha, it's hard to support your duties or aspirations.
- Without Kama, life can become dry and mechanical.
- Without Moksha, all other pursuits feel incomplete.

So happiness blossoms when life flows through all four —

- Right living (Dharma) gives direction,
- Right earning (Artha) gives stability,
- Right enjoyment (Kama) gives sweetness, and
- Right awareness (Moksha) gives freedom.

THE FOUR RIVERS

Dharma — the River of Right Living
Flow with truth, act with compassion,
let your duty become devotion.
When your heart and actions align,
peace takes root —
the kind that no storm can shake.

Artha — the River of Right Earning
Create, build, and nourish.
Let your hands be instruments of purpose, not greed.
Wealth that serves life becomes sacred —
a means to uplift, not possess.

Kama — the River of Right Enjoyment
Love the fragrance of the moment,
but don't be lost in its bloom.
Taste the beauty of art, music, touch, and laughter,
as offerings to the Divine within all.
Pleasure turns to joy
when the heart remains free.

Moksha — the River of Liberation
When the mind grows silent,
and the "I" dissolves into the Infinite,
you realize —
you were never bound, never incomplete.
The joy you sought was your own reflection
in every wave of life.

And so the four rivers unite,
merging in the ocean of Being —
where purpose becomes peace,
and living itself becomes a prayer.

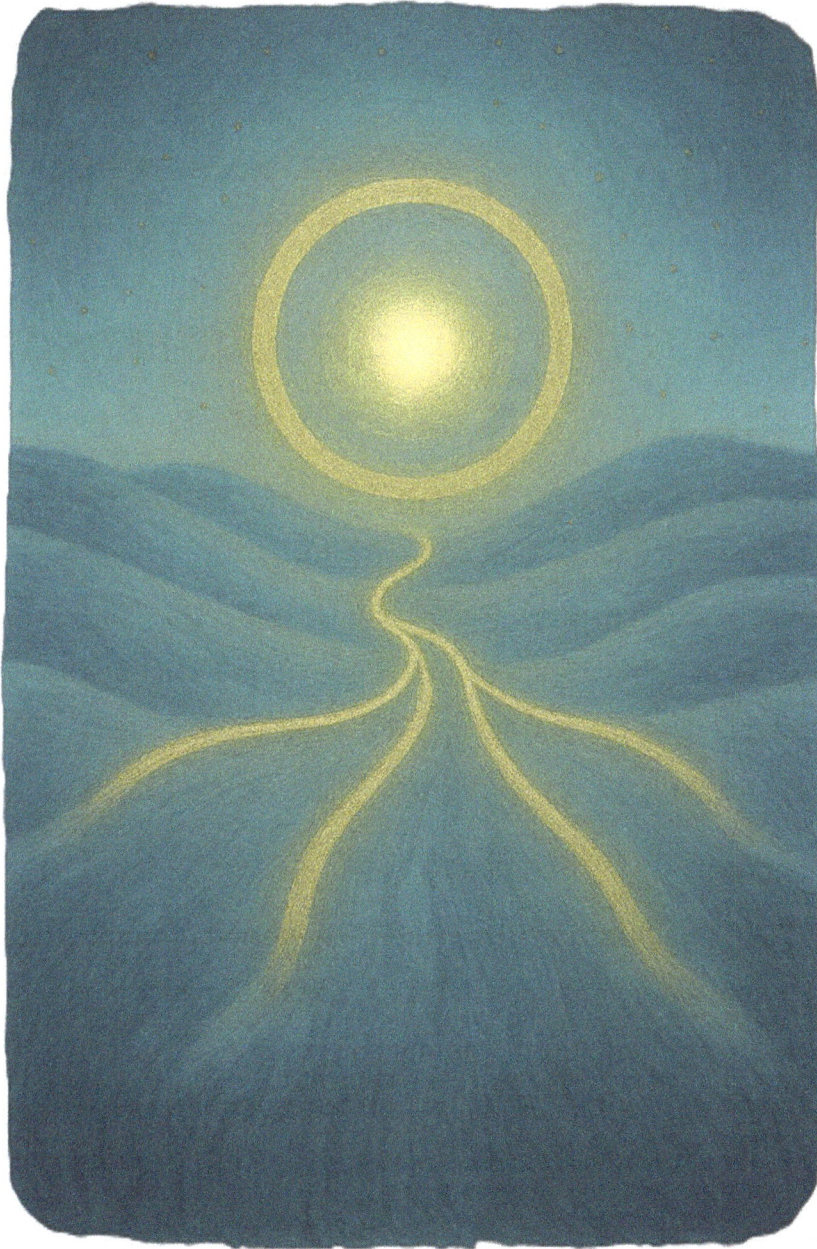

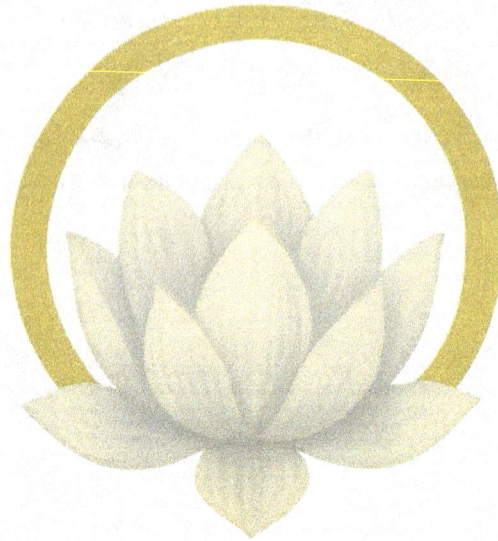

DHARMA — THE PATH OF RIGHTEOUS LIVING

MEANING OF DHARMA

The word Dharma comes from the Sanskrit root "dhṛ", meaning to hold, sustain, or uphold. It is that which holds the universe together — the unseen order that sustains harmony in life, society, and nature.

In simple terms, Dharma is the right way of living — doing what is true, just, and aligned with your inner nature (Swadharma) and the universal good.

LEVELS OF DHARMA

1. **Universal Dharma (Sanatana Dharma):** The eternal principles that apply to all — truth, non-violence, compassion, honesty, purity, patience, and self-control. These are like the laws of nature for the human spirit.

2. **Social Dharma:** The duties we uphold in our relationships — as a friend, parent, teacher, citizen, or leader. It's about acting responsibly within your role, bringing harmony to the collective.

3. **Personal Dharma (Swadharma):** This is your unique path — the way your talents, temperament, and purpose express divine order. To live your Swadharma is to honor your true calling without comparing yourself to others.

DHARMA AND HAPPINESS

When you live by Dharma, you live in alignment with truth — and that alignment brings inner peace. Even amidst challenges, your mind remains clear, because your conscience is pure. Dharma leads to joy because it connects you to your higher self. You no longer chase temporary pleasures — you radiate quiet fulfillment born of integrity.

ANCIENT WISDOM ON DHARMA

- Bhagavad Gita (3.35): "Better is one's own Dharma, though imperfectly performed, than the Dharma of another, well performed."
- Manusmriti: "Ahimsa (non-violence), Satya (truth), Asteya (non-stealing), Shauch (purity), Indriya-nigraha (control of senses) — these form the essence of Dharma."

STORY: YUDHISHTHIRA AND THE YAKSHA (MAHABHARATA)

During exile, Yudhishthira and his brothers were dying of thirst. When they found a lake, a Yaksha (divine being) challenged them — anyone who drank before answering his questions would die. The brothers ignored him and fell unconscious, but Yudhishthira listened patiently and answered each question about truth, duty, and righteousness. Impressed by his wisdom and humility, the Yaksha revealed himself as Dharma, his divine father, and revived the brothers.

Teaching: Dharma is patience, integrity, and listening to conscience even in crisis. When one acts with righteousness, protection and peace arise naturally.

THE ESSENCE OF DHARMA

Dharma is not just about duty or righteousness — it is the innate nature of our being, the truth of who we are when we are fully aligned with the Self. Just as the dharma of sugar is sweetness, the dharma of fire is to give warmth and light, the dharma of a river is to flow, so too, our dharma as human beings is to express the divine qualities that dwell within us.

THE CIRCLE OF LIFE AND LIBERATION

Life begins with curiosity (Brahmacharya),

flowers into creativity (Gṛhastha),

matures into contemplation (Vānaprastha),

and culminates in liberation (Sannyāsa).

Throughout this sacred journey, happiness changes its form —

from outer pleasure to inner peace,

from doing to being,

from seeking to shining.

When Dharma guides every stage,

when Artha and Kāma serve, not enslave,

and when Moksha illumines all,

life itself becomes Yajña — a sacred offering of bliss to the Divine.

THE INQUIRY — "WHO AM I?"

Before understanding Dharma, one must ask:

Who am I?

Am I this body, bound by senses and form?

Am I this prāṇa, that sustains life?

Am I this mind, full of thoughts and desires?

Or am I the intellect that discerns right from wrong?

When this inquiry deepens, realization dawns —

I am not just body, mind, or intellect.

I am the Ātman,

the embodiment of Love (Prema Swaroopa),

the essence of Peace (Shānti Swaroopa),

and the source of Bliss (Ānanda Swaroopa).

TO LIVE ONE'S DHARMA

When I know this truth,
then to live my Dharma means
to act, speak, and think in harmony with my true nature.

If I am Prema Swaroopa,
then my thoughts and actions must radiate love.

If I am Shānti Swaroopa,
then I must cultivate calmness amidst chaos.

If I am Ānanda Swaroopa,
then I must share joy, not sorrow, wherever I go.

Thus, Dharma is not a commandment —
it is a remembrance.

It is the art of being what you truly are.

IN SIMPLE WORDS

When sugar forgets its sweetness,
it cannot be itself.

When the soul forgets its bliss,
it lives in confusion.

To remember your nature is Dharma —
to live it, is Yoga.

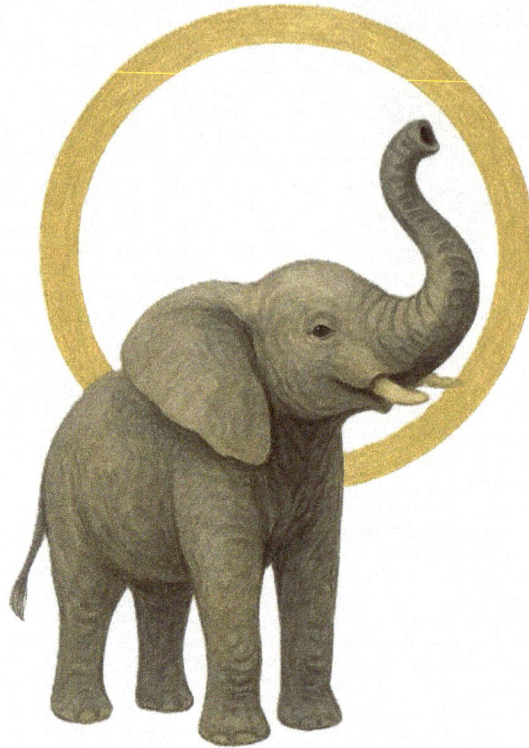

ARTHA — THE PATH OF RIGHTFUL PROSPERITY

MEANING OF ARTHA

In Sanskrit, Artha means "means, purpose, or wealth." It represents the material foundation of life — the resources, skills, and structures we need to live with dignity and to fulfill our Dharma (righteous duties).

Artha includes:

- Wealth and possessions earned ethically
- Education and knowledge as means to sustain life
- Career, livelihood, and social security
- The ability to provide for family, society, and oneself

So, Artha is not greed — it's grounded prosperity. It's the art of creating abundance while staying rooted in ethics and compassion.

SPIRITUAL PERSPECTIVE

The Vedas and Upanishads never rejected material life — they saw it as a sacred expression of divine energy. Money, land, and prosperity (Lakshmi) were considered holy when earned through Dharma and used with gratitude. In this sense, Artha is sacred when it serves life. When wealth is used to support education, charity, healing, art, and community, it becomes Yajna — a sacred offering to society.

ARTHA AND HAPPINESS

Artha brings a sense of stability, confidence, and freedom from fear. When your basic needs are met, your mind becomes calm, ready to pursue higher joys like Kama (creative pleasure) and Moksha (spiritual growth).

However — When Artha is pursued without Dharma, it leads to stress, greed, and imbalance. But when it is pursued with Dharma, it brings contentment, generosity, and gratitude.

So the Vedic wisdom is clear: "Earn righteously. Enjoy mindfully. Share generously."

PRACTICAL WAYS TO LIVE ARTHA

- Choose a profession that aligns with your Swadharma (inner calling).
- Earn with honesty and respect for others' well-being.
- Manage resources mindfully — wealth is energy, not ego.
- Share — through charity, teaching, or service.
- Express gratitude for what you have before asking for more.

Artha is the grounding energy of life — it gives structure to dreams, strength to Dharma, and stability to love. When balanced, it transforms wealth into well-being, and work into worship.

STORY: KING JANAKA'S WEALTH AND DETACHMENT (UPANISHADIC LORE)

King Janaka was both a ruler and a sage. He lived amidst wealth, palaces, and luxury — yet remained inwardly free. When his palace once caught fire, he calmly said, "Nothing of mine is burning." His mind was so rooted in awareness that he saw the world as divine play. Sages came to test him, but found that his prosperity did not enslave him — it expressed his Dharma.

Teaching: True Artha is earned and used with awareness. Wealth is sacred when it serves life, learning, and upliftment — not ego. Janaka shows how one can be "in the world, yet not of it. Artha not just as "wealth" or "prosperity," but as a purposeful manifestation of divine energy in the world — aligned with your true Self, your Swaroopa.

THE ESSENCE OF ARTHA

In ordinary terms, Artha means wealth, resources, and means of living. But in the deeper Vedic vision, Artha means "that which gives meaning, value, and support to life."

The Sanskrit root "Arth" means purpose, meaning, or essence. So, Artha is not only what you possess, but what you live for.

ARTHA AND DHARMA — THE INNER CONNECTION

When Dharma (your true nature) is understood, Artha becomes the outer expression of that inner truth. If Dharma is who you are, then Artha is how you manifest it in the world.

- If your Dharma is love (Prema Swaroopa), your Artha becomes creating spaces, relationships, and works that spread love.
- If your Dharma is peace (Shānti Swaroopa), your Artha becomes creating harmony — in your home, your work, your environment.
- If your Dharma is bliss (Ānanda Swaroopa), your Artha becomes sharing joy, wisdom, or healing through whatever path life gives you.

ARTHA AS ENERGY, NOT POSSESSION

In the Vedic view, wealth is sacred energy (Lakshmi). It is not to be hoarded, but to flow in dharmic ways. It nourishes, uplifts, and sustains — when aligned with higher purpose. So, Artha includes:

- Physical resources and livelihood
- Knowledge and skills
- Relationships and goodwill
- Creative potential
- Spiritual merit (Punya)

All of these are forms of Lakshmi — divine abundance — meant to serve Dharma.

THE VEDIC FORMULA OF ARTHA

- When Dharma guides Artha, it becomes a blessing.
- When Desire (Kāma) drives Artha, it becomes bondage.
- When Awareness (Moksha) illumines Artha, it becomes pure energy flowing through divine hands.

IN SIMPLE WORDS

Artha is not the gold you hold,
but the light you unfold.

It is the material reflection
of your inner abundance.

When your work, wealth, and creations
arise from love and awareness,
your Artha becomes sacred —
your life, an offering.

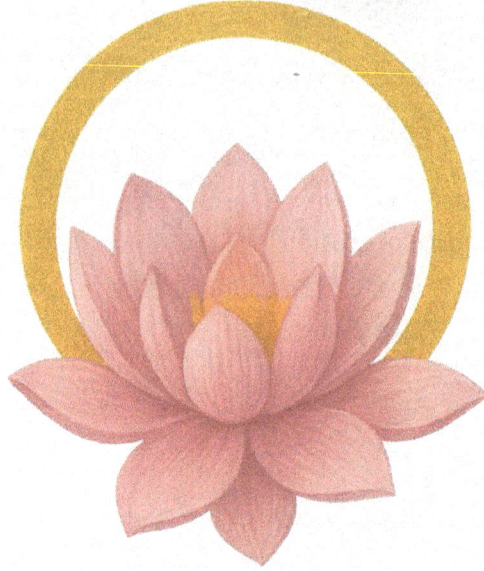

KAMA — THE PATH OF LOVE AND BEAUTY

MEANING OF KĀMA

In Sanskrit, Kāma means desire, love, or pleasure — not only sensual pleasure, but the deep longing for connection, beauty, and joy in all its forms.

It includes:

- Aesthetic joy (art, music, poetry, fragrance, beauty)
- Emotional love (friendship, affection, devotion)
- Sensual and sexual pleasure (expressed with reverence and respect)
- The happiness of a content, expressive, and grateful heart

Kāma is the celebration of life — the sweetness that gives meaning to Dharma and Artha.

SPIRITUAL UNDERSTANDING OF KĀMA

In Vedic philosophy, Kāma is not condemned; it is divine when aligned with Dharma. It becomes sacred when it flows from love, not lust; appreciation, not attachment.

The Rig Veda even describes Kāma as the first creative impulse of the cosmos — "Kāma arose in the beginning, the first seed of mind." It means: the entire universe was born from desire — the desire of the Divine to know Itself through creation.

So, desire itself is not the problem — ignorance is. When desire serves the higher self, it becomes creativity and joy; when it serves the ego, it becomes craving and bondage.

KĀMA AND HAPPINESS

Kāma brings happiness through aesthetic fulfillment and emotional harmony. It softens the heart, opens you to love, and allows you to experience the Divine in all forms of beauty.

Yet — when unbalanced, Kāma leads to overindulgence and restlessness. When balanced by Dharma and awareness, it becomes Rasa — the pure essence of joy that uplifts the soul.

HEALTHY EXPRESSION OF KĀMA

- Appreciating art, music, fragrance, and nature with mindfulness.
- Cultivating loving relationships grounded in respect and truth.
- Enjoying the senses without being enslaved by them.
- Turning personal love into Prema — universal love.
- Seeing beauty as a reflection of the Divine everywhere.

IN ESSENCE

Kāma is the fragrance of existence — it gives color to life, warmth to Dharma, and sweetness to Artha. When purified by awareness, it becomes devotion (Bhakti), when unrestrained by wisdom, it becomes attachment (Moha).

So the Vedic way is not to suppress desire, but to refine it until every joy becomes an offering to the Divine within all things.

STORY: RATI AND KĀMA DEVA (PURĀṆAS)

When Lord Shiva went into deep meditation, the gods sent Kāma Deva (the god of love) to awaken him, so the cosmic creation could continue. Kāma's arrow of desire disturbed Shiva's penance, and Shiva, in anger, opened his third eye and burned Kāma to ashes. Rati, Kāma's wife, wept in grief, and through her deep devotion and pure love, Shiva was moved, and in fact, the Goddess Parvati recreated him from his ashes and restored Kāmadev to life — but without a body, as Ananga (formless love). Kamadeva and Ananga are two forms of the Hindu god of love and desire. Kamadeva is a personified deity with a physical body, but after Shiva incinerated him, he was reborn as Ananga, the "bodiless one," symbolizing love's existence beyond physical form. Ananga represents the enduring, intangible aspect of love, passion, and longing that fills the cosmos even without a physical body.

Teaching: Desire (Kāma) has two faces — when it serves creation and love, it uplifts; when it disturbs awareness, it binds. Purified by devotion (Rati's love), desire becomes divine — Kāma without form, love without attachment.

KĀMA, THE MOST OFTEN MISUNDERSTOOD OF THE PURUSHARTHAS

If Dharma is the truth of your being, and Artha is the manifestation of that truth in the world, then Kāma is the joy of experiencing and celebrating that manifestation.

In Sanskrit, Kāma means desire, love, beauty, and sensory enjoyment. But in the Vedic vision, it is much more sacred — it is the creative pulse of life itself.

The universe was born from Kāma. In the Rig Veda (10.129), it is said: "In the beginning, desire (Kāma) arose in the One — it was the first seed of the mind."

So, Kāma is not sin — it is the divine longing of creation to know itself, the cosmic impulse of Love seeking expression.

TRUE KĀMA VS. WORLDLY CRAVING

When Kāma is guided by Dharma, it becomes devotion, beauty, art, compassion, and union. When Kāma loses Dharma, it becomes craving, attachment, and suffering. So, true Kāma is not lust or greed, but the joyful participation in the dance of life — through love, music, touch, beauty, and creativity — while remaining rooted in awareness.

KĀMA AND THE SENSES

Our senses (Indriyas) are instruments of delight — but the sage enjoys through them without being enslaved by them.

- To see beauty and recognize the Divine in it — is Kāma refined by Dharma.
- To hear music and feel your soul expand — is Kāma sanctified by awareness.
- To love another and awaken to your shared divinity — is Kāma as Yoga.

Thus, Kāma becomes a path of Bhakti — the art of finding God through beauty and love.

KĀMA IN HUMAN LIFE

Kāma gives meaning to our emotions — it allows joy, affection, friendship, art, and romance to flower. It keeps life fragrant and heart-centered. But like fire, Kāma must be tended with reverence. When disciplined by Dharma and balanced by Artha, it becomes a sacred flame — not a wildfire.

IN SIMPLE WORDS

Kāma is the sweetness of life
experienced through awakened senses.
It is the divine desire to love, create, and connect.

When guided by Dharma and expressed through Artha,
Kāma becomes worship —
and the heart becomes a temple of joy.

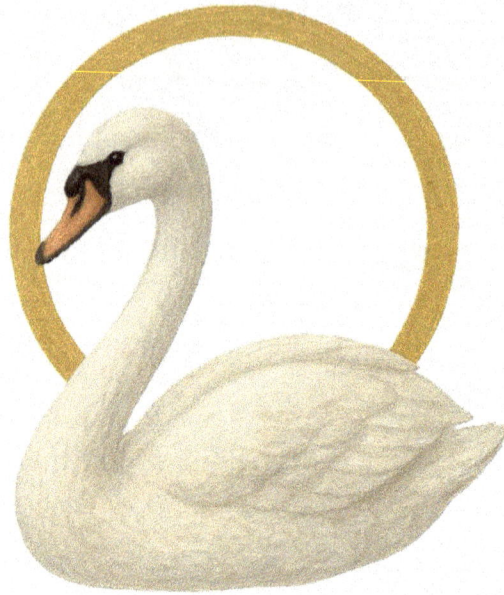

MOKSHA — THE PATH OF LIBERATION

MEANING OF MOKSHA

Moksha means freedom, release, or liberation — freedom from all bondage of the mind, ego, and illusion (Maya). It is the realization that you are not the limited body or mind, but the infinite consciousness (Atman) — pure, eternal, and untouched by suffering.

While Dharma, Artha, and Kāma help us live gracefully in the world, Moksha is awakening from the world's illusion, realizing that joy, peace, and truth were never outside — they were always you.

THE ESSENCE OF MOKSHA

Moksha is not escapism or renunciation of life. It is freedom while living (Jivanmukti) — a state of inner peace, even amidst change, because you have realized: "I am not the doer, not the sufferer, not the seeker — I am the witness, the eternal Self."

When you awaken to that truth, fear, anger, and desire lose their grip. You live fully, love deeply, but remain inwardly free.

HOW MOKSHA ARISES

Moksha is attained through Self-knowledge (Jnana) and awareness. It unfolds through:

- Meditation and silence — realizing the stillness beneath all noise.
- Detachment (Vairagya) — enjoying without clinging.
- Selfless action (Karma Yoga) — acting without expectation.
- Devotion (Bhakti) — surrendering the "I" into Divine Love.
- Inquiry (Jnana Yoga) — asking, Who am I? until all illusion falls away.

In truth, Moksha is not something to gain — it's the recognition of what you already are.

MOKSHA AND HAPPINESS

Moksha brings the highest joy — Ānanda. Not the fleeting happiness of outer achievements, but the bliss of being whole. In this state:

- You see yourself in all beings and all beings in yourself.
- You live without fear of death or loss.
- You experience compassion without effort.
- You rest in peace that no external situation can disturb.

It is the freedom of the ocean that no longer identifies with the waves. Moksha is the flowering of consciousness. Where Dharma gives direction, Artha gives stability, and Kāma gives sweetness — Moksha gives meaning to it all.

STORY: NACHIKETA AND YAMA (KATHA UPANISHAD)

The young seeker Nachiketa questioned his father's false ritual offerings and was sent to the abode of Yama, the god of death. Fearless and pure, Nachiketa waited three days without food until Yama returned. Impressed, Yama offered him three boons. Nachiketa asked first for his father's peace, second for knowledge of sacred fire, and third — the secret of what lies beyond death. Yama tested him, offering wealth and pleasures instead, but Nachiketa refused. He said, "All pleasures fade, O Death — tell me that which is eternal." Yama, pleased, revealed the truth of the immortal Self (Atman) — and Nachiketa attained liberation.

Teaching: Moksha is the awakening that comes when one seeks the eternal beyond the fleeting. Freedom is found not by running away from life, but by seeing through its illusions.

SHORT REFLECTION

When the mind grows silent,
and desire turns to devotion,
the walls of "I" and "mine" dissolve.

What remains is freedom —
the simple joy of being.
This is Moksha.

THE JOURNEY OF PURUSHARTHA – FROM PURPOSE TO LIBERATION

In the beginning,
a whisper arises in the heart —
"Why am I here?"

And the soul, ancient and patient, answers:
"There are four rivers that flow toward wholeness —
walk them with awareness, and you shall return to yourself."

THE ESSENCE OF MOKSHA

Moksha in Sanskrit means liberation, release, or freedom. But not freedom from life — rather, freedom within life. It is not about escaping the world; it is about awakening in the world.

It is the deep peace that dawns when the soul remembers:
"I am not bound by this body,
not trapped in the mind,
not limited by birth or death.
I am pure awareness — Sat, Chit, Ānanda —
existence, consciousness, and bliss."

WHAT ARE WE LIBERATED FROM?

Not from the world — but from illusion (Māyā).

Not from relationships — but from attachment.

Not from karma — but from identification with the doer.

When one awakens to their eternal Self, they realize: "Nothing ever truly bound me.
I was the sky, watching the clouds all along."

This realization is Moksha — the stillness beyond striving, the joy beyond desire, the peace beyond opposites.

MOKSHA IN DAILY LIFE

Moksha is not just a final event after death — it can be lived moment by moment. Whenever you act without ego, love without condition, and rest in awareness — you are already free. Freedom is not something gained; it is something remembered.

IN SIMPLE WORDS

Moksha is not a destination — it is awakening. It is the silence between two thoughts, the love behind all forms, the smile of the soul when it recognizes itself.

It is freedom from becoming, and rest in being.

THE CIRCLE COMPLETE

Dharma teaches you who you are.

Artha shows you what you can create.

Kāma lets you taste the beauty of existence.

Moksha reveals that you were always whole —
untouched, infinite, and free.

And thus the journey of happiness,
the teaching of the Bhrigu Valli,
and the wisdom of the Vedas
merge into one eternal truth:

"Ānando Brahma — Bliss is the nature of the Divine."

THE FOUR PURUSHARTHAS FULFILLED

When Dharma is lived truthfully,
Artha earned righteously,
and Kāma enjoyed consciously —
then Moksha arises naturally.

It is the flower of a well-lived, well-loved life.

Not renunciation of the world, but realization of the Self within it.

THE VEDIC PATH

Dharma gives direction,
Artha gives stability,
Kāma gives sweetness,
and Moksha gives freedom.

Together, they form the complete circle of happiness —
where desire serves purpose,
purpose serves truth,
and truth reveals bliss.

Dharma - The River of Truth
Walk with integrity, child of light.
Let your thoughts be clear,
your actions kind,
your choices rooted in compassion.
When your life becomes aligned with truth,
peace flowers in your heart like morning sun —
gentle, steadfast, unshakable.

Artha - The River of Purpose
Build with care, earn with grace.
Let your work be an offering,
not a chase.
Prosperity that uplifts is holy —
when wealth becomes service,
and effort becomes prayer.
Then abundance flows,
not as possession, but as blessing

Kāma – The River of Beauty

Rejoice in the fragrance of life —

in music, in touch, in art, in love.

Let desire be a doorway to devotion,

not a chain of craving.

Savor each moment as divine nectar,

for every joy, when blessed by awareness,

becomes a hymn to the Beloved.

Moksha – The River of Freedom

And when all rivers merge within,

you awaken —

not as the seeker,

but as the ocean itself.

The "I" dissolves into stillness,

and only Being remains —

silent, infinite, radiant.

No more to seek, no more to strive,only to be.

The Four Rivers Flow as One

Dharma gives direction,

Artha gives strength,

Kāma gives sweetness,

Moksha gives peace.

Together, they form the sacred circle of life —

where living becomes prayer,

and every breath sings,

"I am whole."

THE HARMONY OF THE FOUR

- Dharma guides your actions.
- Artha sustains your responsibilities.
- Kāma sweetens your journey.
- Moksha frees your spirit.

Together, they form the complete human experience — where you live with virtue, create with purpose, love with depth, and awaken with peace.

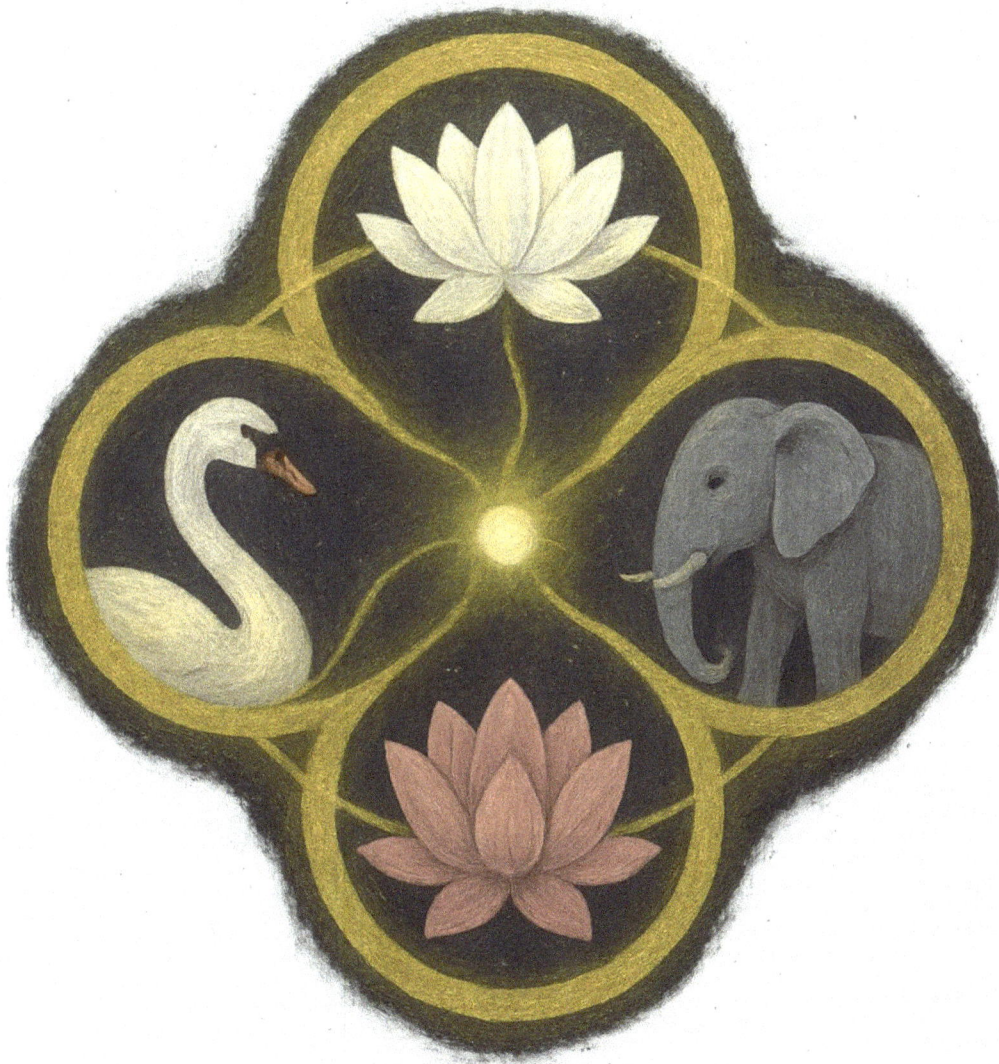

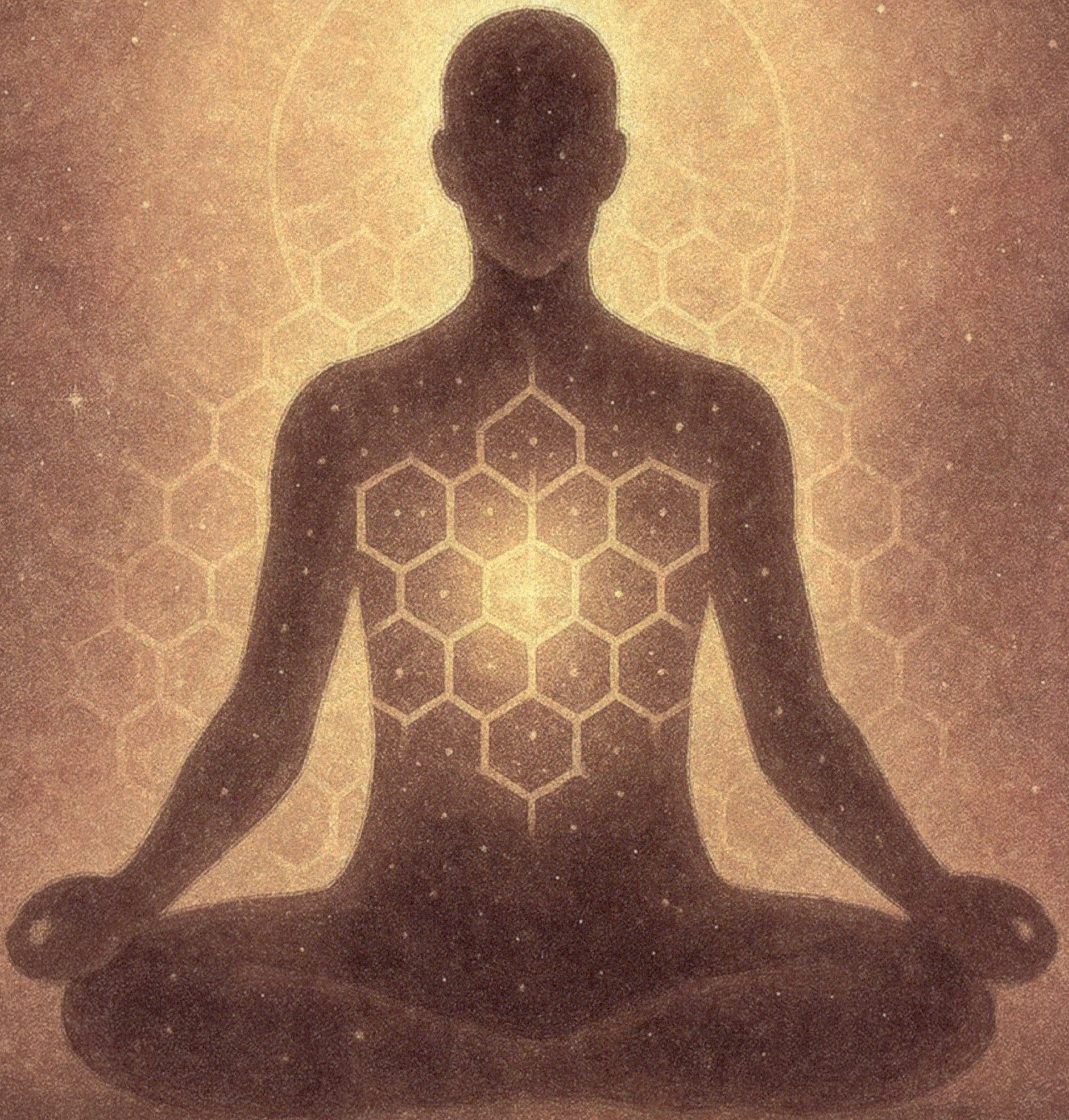

BHRIGU VALLI

The Bhrigu Valli of the Taittiriya Upanishad is indeed one of the most exquisite revelations of Vedic wisdom on happiness (Ānanda). It beautifully describes how the sage Bhrigu, guided by his teacher and father Varuna, embarks on a deep inner inquiry into the source of true happiness. This journey, known as the "Ānanda Mimamsa" — the Inquiry into Bliss, is one of the most poetic and profound teachings in all the Upanishads.

THE STORY — THE INQUIRY OF BHRIGU

The young sage Bhrigu approaches his father Varuna, asking: "Revered Sir, what is Brahman (the ultimate reality)?"

Varuna replies: "From whom all beings are born, by whom they live, and into whom they return — that is Brahman."

He instructs Bhrigu to meditate and realize this truth through contemplation (tapas). Bhrigu begins his journey inward — stage by stage — discovering what truly sustains and fulfills life.

THE FIVE SHEATHS OF EXPERIENCE (PANCHA-KOSHA VIVEKA)

Bhrigu realizes that life is sustained through layers — each more subtle and real than the previous. Through meditation, he discovers that happiness deepens as consciousness moves inward from the gross to the subtle.

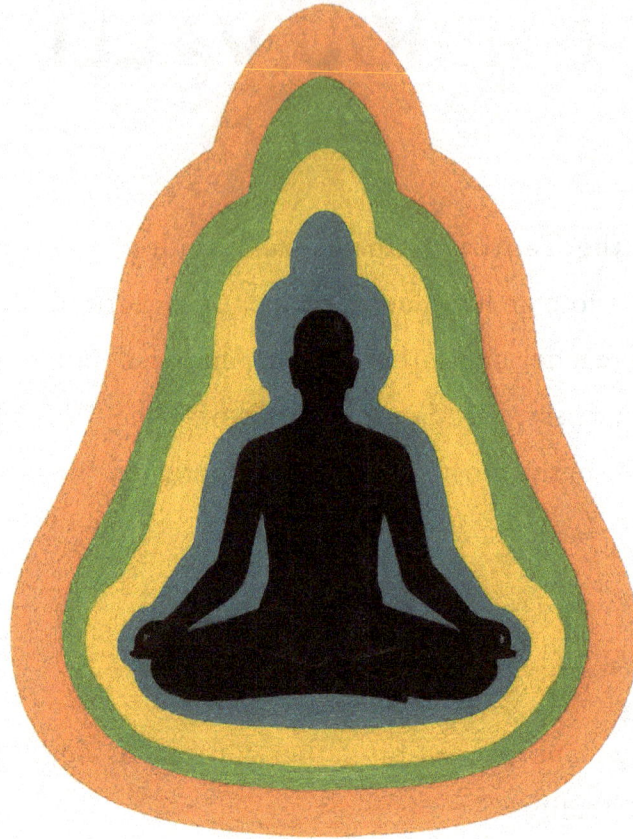

1. Annamaya Kosha – The Food Sheath

- He first perceives: From food, beings are born; by food they live; into food they return.

- He concludes: Food is Brahman.

- But later he realizes — this is limited happiness, dependent on the senses.

2. Prāṇamaya Kosha – The Vital Energy Sheath

- Meditating deeper, he discovers: The life-force (prāṇa) sustains food, perception, and action.

- He experiences joy in vitality, but still feels — this too passes.

3. Manomaya Kosha – The Mental Sheath

- Going deeper, he experiences: The mind organizes the world of thoughts, desires, and experiences.

- Joy from understanding and creativity is higher, yet still fluctuates.

4. Vijñānamaya Kosha – The Wisdom Sheath

- Further meditating, Bhrigu realizes the joy of discernment and awareness — when one acts from clarity and truth.
- Yet, even this wisdom has boundaries — it knows, but does not become.

5. Ānandamaya Kosha – The Bliss Sheath

- Finally, through profound silence, Bhrigu enters Ānanda — the pure joy that has no cause, no object, no end.
- Here, he realizes: Ānanda is Brahman — from Bliss all beings are born, by Bliss they live, and into Bliss they return.

VEDIC UNDERSTANDING OF HAPPINESS

From Bhrigu Valli, we learn: True happiness (Ānanda) is not sensory pleasure (Kāma), not success (Artha), and not even intellectual pride (Vijñāna). It is the essence of existence itself — the bliss of being in tune with the Self (Ātman). Everything else — food, vitality, mind, intellect — are expressions of that one Bliss. This is why the Upanishad declares: "Ānando Brahmeti Vyajānāt — He realized that Bliss is Brahman."

THE WISDOM IN SIMPLE WORDS

Bhrigu's journey shows that:

- Outer joy begins with nourishment (food and vitality).
- Inner joy deepens with awareness (mind and understanding).
- True joy blossoms in realization (Ānanda) — when you rest in your true nature.

So the Vedic formula of happiness is not "to seek" joy, but to uncover it — layer by layer — until the bliss of being shines naturally.

THE JOURNEY OF BHRIGU

Bhrigu sat in silence,
listening to the breath of creation.

He tasted the joy of food,
the power of breath,
the music of the mind,
the light of wisdom —
yet none were complete.

Then, in stillness,
he entered the heart's center —
where Bliss itself dwells,
silent, vast, eternal.

There, no hunger, no seeking,
no division remained.

Only Ānanda —
the song of the Self,
echoing through all creation.

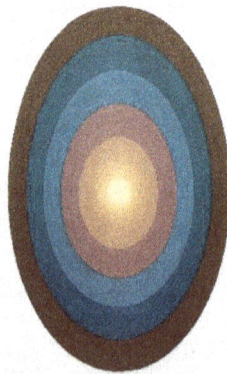

ANNAMAYA KOSHA (THE FOOD SHEATH)

"I am the body made of food — nourished by Earth."

- **Represents:** The physical body composed of the five elements (Pancha Mahabhutas).
- **Nourished by:** Food (Anna), water, and breath.
- Dominated by: Tamas (inertia, matter).
- **Function:** To provide structure, movement, and sensory experience.
- **Realization:** This body is sacred — a temple for the Divine Self.

PRĀNAMAYA KOSHA (THE VITAL SHEATH)

MEANING

"Prāna" means life-force — the subtle energy that animates every living being. This kosha is made up of Prāna, Apāna, Samāna, Udāna, and Vyāna — the five vital winds (Pancha Prānas) that sustain and move the body.

If Annamaya Kosha is the structure, then Prānamaya Kosha is the electric current that makes it come alive.

VEDIC UNDERSTANDING

This sheath connects the physical body with the mind. It governs breathing, circulation, digestion, movement, and vitality. Through it, the subtle energy of life flows — linking body and consciousness. When Prāna is balanced, the body glows with vitality, the mind feels calm, and the heart beats in rhythm with nature.

But when Prāna is disturbed, life feels fragmented — fatigue, anxiety, or imbalance arise. Hence, ancient sages developed Prānāyāma — conscious breathwork — to purify and harmonize this sheath.

- Element: Air (Vāyu)
- Energy Center: Heart (Anāhata Chakra)
- Function: Vitality, health, rhythm of life
- State of Being: Flow and balance

MANOMAYA KOSHA (THE MENTAL–EMOTIONAL SHEATH)

MEANING

The Sanskrit word "Manas" means mind — the seat of thoughts, emotions, imagination, and sensory interpretation. This kosha is subtler than breath (Prānamaya), yet denser than wisdom (Vijñānamaya). It is the layer through which we perceive, react, and feel.

NATURE OF MANOMAYA KOSHA

This sheath receives information from the senses and colors it with our likes, dislikes, fears, desires, and memories. It creates the inner chatter, the stories we tell ourselves — forming the egoic personality.

When the mind is restless, it projects confusion onto life. When it is pure and calm, it reflects the light of the Self clearly — like a still lake reflecting the moon.

HOW IT WORKS

The Manomaya is where our thoughts shape emotions, and emotions shape our reality.

- The five senses (jnanendriyas) feed it information.
- The Prānamaya Kosha energizes it.
- The Vijñānamaya Kosha (next layer) guides it through discernment and wisdom.

DISTURBANCE IN THIS KOSHA

These arise when the mind dominates without the guidance of higher awareness.

- Overthinking and anxiety
- Emotional swings and attachment
- Sleep disturbances
- Fatigue from mental clutter

HEALING AND BALANCING PRACTICES

1. Meditation & Mindfulness — observing thoughts without judgment.
2. Japa or Mantra Chanting — harmonizes the mental vibrations.
3. Satsang (company of truth) — uplifts emotional energy.
4. Writing / Reflection — expressing emotions brings clarity.
5. Nature immersion — trees, rivers, and silence restore mental peace.

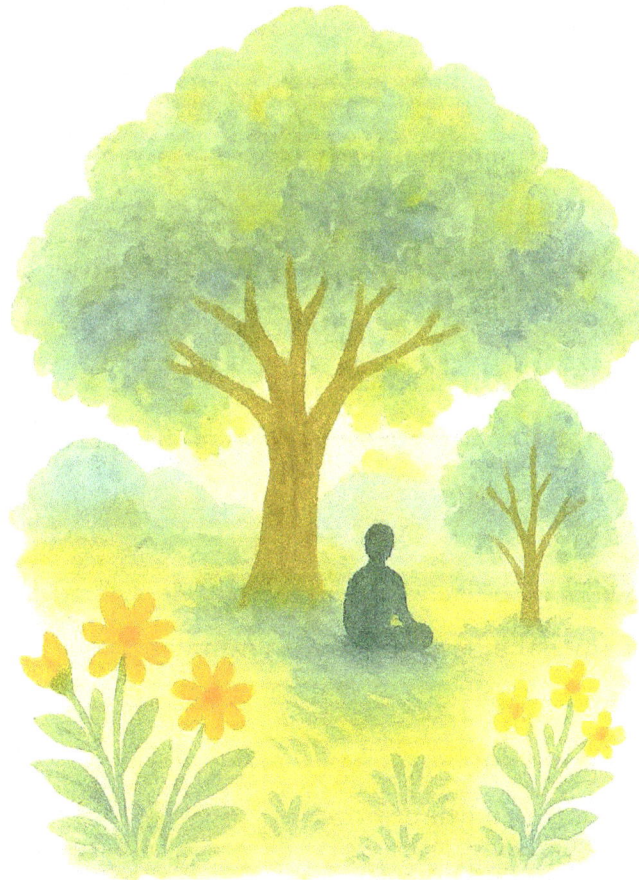

VIJÑĀNAMAYA KOSHA — THE WISDOM SHEATH

MEANING

The Sanskrit word Vijñāna means higher knowledge, insight, or discriminative intelligence — the capacity to perceive reality beyond emotion or thought. It is the sheath of the Buddhi (intellect) and Ahamkara (the sense of "I"). This layer allows us to discern truth from illusion, right from wrong, the eternal from the transient.

NATURE OF VIJÑĀNAMAYA KOSHA

If the Manomaya Kosha is the ocean of thoughts and feelings, the Vijñānamaya Kosha is the light that guides the ship safely across. It holds our values, beliefs, intuition, ethics, and spiritual insight — the inner compass that aligns us with our dharma and higher purpose. When this sheath awakens, life ceases to be mechanical and becomes meaningful. We begin to act from wisdom, not reaction; from clarity, not confusion.

FUNCTION

It transforms mental information into living wisdom — just as sunlight transforms a seed into a flower.

- Integrates knowledge (jnāna) with experience (anubhava).
- Directs the mind through discrimination (viveka).
- Aligns daily life with spiritual truth.
- Recognizes the Self behind the personality.

WHEN IMBALANCED

A clouded intellect becomes the barrier between mind and soul.

- Confusion about purpose
- Inner conflict or moral doubt
- Over-intellectualization without heart
- Blind belief without inquiry

46

HEALING AND BALANCING PRACTICES

1. Svādhyāya (self-study) — reading and reflecting on sacred texts.
2. Contemplation & silence — letting wisdom ripen naturally.
3. Satsang — company of evolved souls that uplift consciousness.
4. Karma Yoga — selfless service purifies the ego.
5. Meditation on the Witness — observing thoughts without identity.

ĀNANDAMAYA KOSHA — THE BLISS SHEATH

MEANING

The word Ānanda means bliss, joy, delight, or eternal contentment. Ānandamaya Kosha literally translates to "that which is made of bliss." This sheath is not about emotional pleasure or sensory happiness — it is the innate serenity of the Self that shines when all other layers fall silent. It is not something to be achieved, but rather revealed, when the mind, intellect, and body rest in harmony.

NATURE OF ĀNANDAMAYA KOSHA

This is the subtlest veil before pure consciousness (Ātman). It is the still, luminous center that remains untouched by joy or sorrow, gain or loss.

In deep meditation or dreamless sleep, you touch this layer — that peaceful, contented silence where you simply are.

STATE OF BEING

This is where one says: "I am not seeking peace — I am peace."

- No striving, no thought — just being.
- A feeling of wholeness, contentment, and love without reason.
- Unity — not between opposites, but beyond them

VEDIC UNDERSTANDING

"Ānando brahmeti vyajānāt"

(He realized: Bliss is Brahman.)

— *Taittirīya Upaniṣad*

In the Taittirīya Upaniṣad (Bhrigu Valli), the seeker Bhrigu ascends through all the koshas — food, prāna, mind, intellect — and finally realizes that Ānanda (bliss) is the true nature of Brahman. This means the essence of existence itself is bliss — not fleeting joy, but infinite stillness filled with divine love.

WHEN AWAKENED

- Unshakable inner peace
- Compassion and effortless kindness
- Gratitude toward all life
- Spontaneous joy that radiates to others

WAYS TO AWAKEN THE ĀNANDAMAYA KOSHA

1. Deep Meditation (Dhyāna): Resting in pure awareness beyond thought.
2. Bhakti (Devotion): Surrendering to the Divine with love and trust.
3. Seva (Selfless Service): Expressing bliss through compassionate action.
4. Satsang & Silence: Absorbing truth in presence of higher consciousness.
5. Gratitude Practice: Seeing every moment as divine grace.

SYMBOLISM

- Element: Ether (Ākāśa) — boundless and pure
- Chakra Association: Sahasrāra (Crown)
- State of Being: Pure bliss, unity, and self-realization
- Function: Reveals the presence of the Self behind all experience

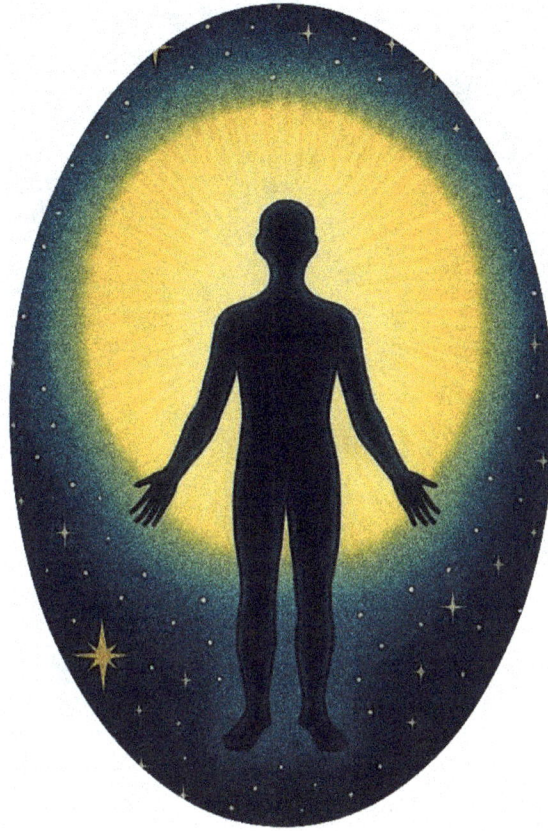

ESSENCE

When all other koshas — body, breath, mind, and intellect — are quiet and balanced, the Ānandamaya Kosha shines naturally, like the sun behind passing clouds.

This is the source of true happiness — not from doing or having, but from being what you truly are: Sat-Chit-Ānanda — Existence, Consciousness, Bliss.

VEDIC INSIGHT

"Prāna is the bridge between body and soul."
— *Taittirīya Upaniṣad*

When breath becomes conscious, life itself becomes sacred. When breath flows freely, awareness expands naturally toward peace.

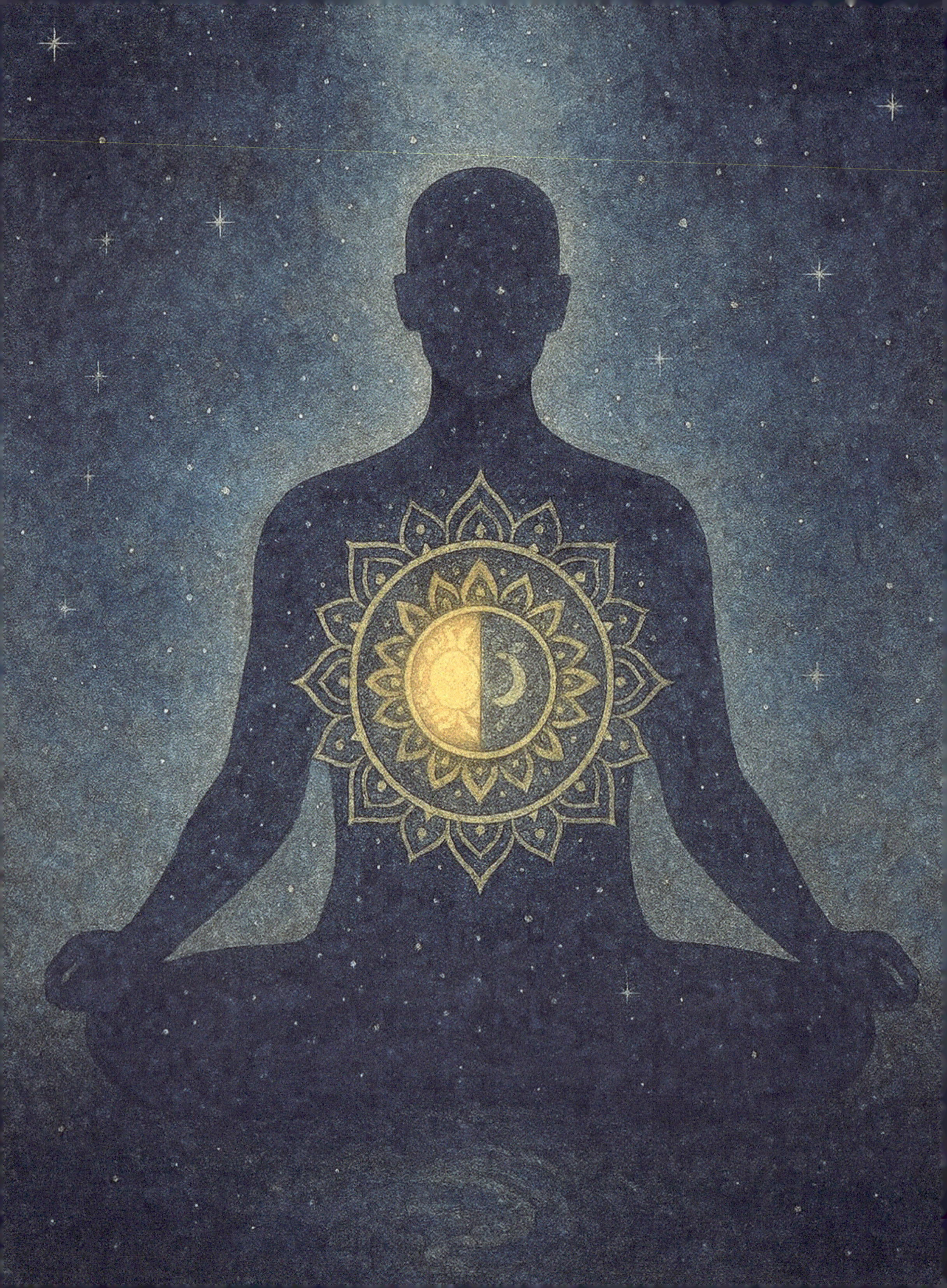

THE SECRET OF HAPPINESS

Bliss is not attained — it is remembered. Each of these techniques is a doorway back to your own infinite nature — where happiness is not pursued, but revealed.

1. THE SACRED PAUSE — AWARENESS BETWEEN BREATHS

"Between two breaths, in the gap, the mystery blossoms."

Essence: Focus on the still point between inhalation and exhalation — that subtle pause where breath stops.

Practice: Inhale deeply... pause... exhale slowly... pause again. In that stillness, awareness awakens.

Wisdom: The breath is life's dance between being and becoming. In the pause, the mind disappears — only consciousness remains.

2. THE FLAME WITHIN — MEDITATION ON INNER LIGHT

"At the heart's center shines a flame — timeless, deathless, divine."

Essence: Close your eyes and visualize a small golden flame in the heart.

Practice: Let the flame expand with each breath, illuminating your entire being.

Wisdom: The inner light is not imagination — it is your true self, the radiant consciousness beyond all shadows.

3. AWARENESS AT THE EDGE OF SLEEP

"When night meets dawn, when wakefulness kisses sleep — that twilight holds the key."

Essence: As you drift into sleep, stay gently aware — that is the doorway to the Infinite.

Practice: Each night, observe the moment you begin to fall asleep. Don't resist, just witness.

Wisdom: Between waking and dreaming lies a sacred silence — the same silence from which creation arises.

4. THE FIRE OF DESIRE — ENTERING THROUGH PASSION

"In the heart of desire, find the spark of divine longing."

Essence: When a deep emotion or desire arises, don't suppress it — dive into its energy with awareness.

Practice: Feel the energy fully, without labeling it as good or bad.

Let it melt into pure aliveness.

Wisdom: All desires are distorted forms of divine love — when seen clearly, they dissolve into bliss.

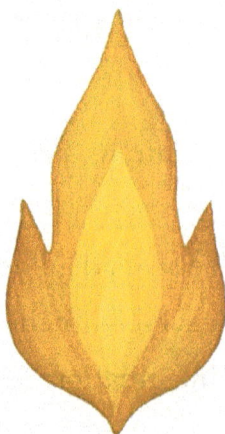

5. LISTENING TO THE INNER SOUND (NĀDA)

"Listen not with ears, but with your being — the unstruck sound sings within."

Essence: There is a subtle hum within you — the soundless sound of existence.

Practice: Sit quietly and listen — beneath all noise, a vibration is always there.

Wisdom: That eternal resonance (Anāhata Nāda) connects you to the heart of creation — where silence and sound are one.

6. THE SKY MEDITATION — BOUNDLESS AWARENESS

"Gaze into the endless sky — and become the sky."

Essence: Look at the open sky without focusing on anything.

Practice: Let your awareness expand into that vastness until inner boundaries dissolve.

Wisdom: You are not the body gazing at the sky — you are the space in which the sky appears.

7. THE TASTE OF PRESENCE

"When you eat or drink, taste fully — it is the flavor of existence."

Essence: Every sensory act can become a doorway to the sacred.

Practice: When eating, drinking, or smelling a flower — be completely aware of the taste, texture, and sensation.

Wisdom: The divine is tasted through life itself; nothing is ordinary when seen through awareness.

8. THE CENTER OF THE HEART — SEAT OF THE SELF

"Enter the lotus of the heart — the shrine of peace."

Essence: Direct your attention gently toward the center of your chest.

Practice: Breathe into the heart space. Feel its warmth, love, and stillness.

Wisdom: All roads of meditation lead to the same heart — where Shiva and Shakti are one.

9. THE GAP BETWEEN THOUGHTS

"Between two thoughts, the Truth waits silently."

Essence: Observe the mind's flow — not the thoughts, but the space between them.

Practice: When a thought ends and before another begins — pause there.

Wisdom: Thoughts are ripples on the surface; awareness is the still depth beneath.

10. THE GAZE OF WONDER — SEEING WITHOUT SEEING

"Look at any object as if for the first time — and it reveals the whole."

Essence: Gaze softly at a flower, flame, or tree — without naming or analyzing it.

Practice: Just look — let the seen and the seer merge.

Wisdom: When perception becomes pure, duality fades — everything becomes divine.

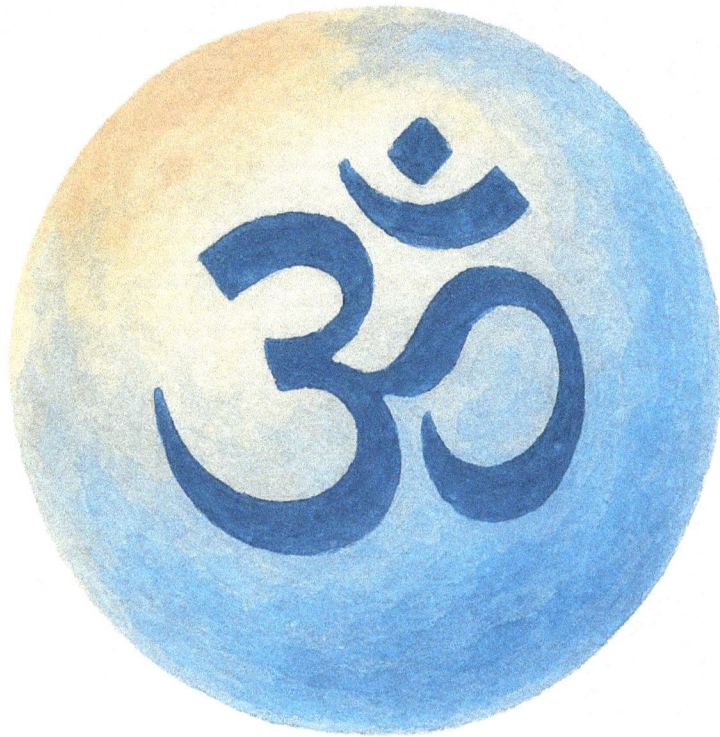

11. THE SOUND OF AUM — RETURNING TO SILENCE

"Chant AUM — let the sound rise and dissolve into silence."

Essence: AUM (ॐ) is the vibration of creation, preservation, and dissolution.

Practice: Chant it slowly — "Aaaa…" "Uuuu…" "Mmmm…" — then rest in the silence after.

Wisdom: The silence after AUM is the heart of Shiva (formless, Nirguna)— pure consciousness, boundless joy.

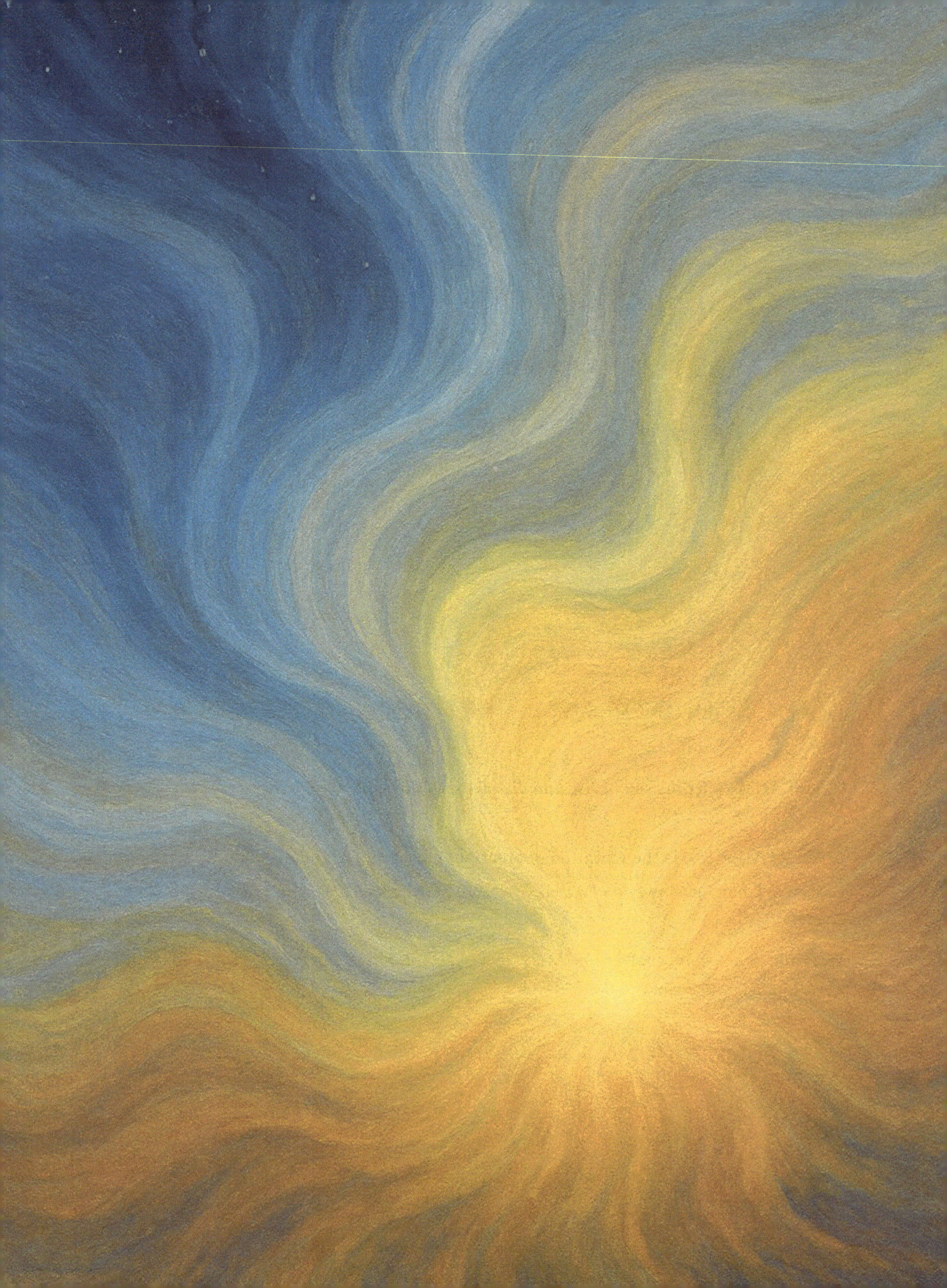

VEDIC VIEW & MODERN SCIENCE OF HAPPINESS HORMONES

The Vedas understood what modern neuroscience is rediscovering today — that our inner chemistry mirrors our consciousness. When we live in tune with Dharma, Nature, and Awareness, the body naturally secretes joy-giving hormones — the Amrita, or "nectar of bliss," described in Upaniṣadic texts.

DOPAMINE — JOY OF PURPOSE AND FULFILLMENT

Vedic Principle: Dharma — Right Action with Awareness

Dopamine = Joy of Progress.

It flows when we live with purpose and alignment — when effort meets meaning.

Vedic Ways to Enhance Dopamine:

1. Morning Brahma Muhurta (4–6 AM): Begin your day with prayer, silence, and gratitude — activating clear purpose.
2. Sankalpa (Sacred Intention): State your daily intention before your morning rituals: "May my actions today serve truth and light."
3. Discipline (Tapas): Keep small daily commitments — yoga, study, meditation. Each completed vow refines dopamine flow.
4. Music & Mantra: Chant uplifting mantras like "Om Shreem Namah" (Lakshmi beej) — aligning effort with grace.

Mantra for Purpose: "Om Tat Sat" — My actions are guided by truth.

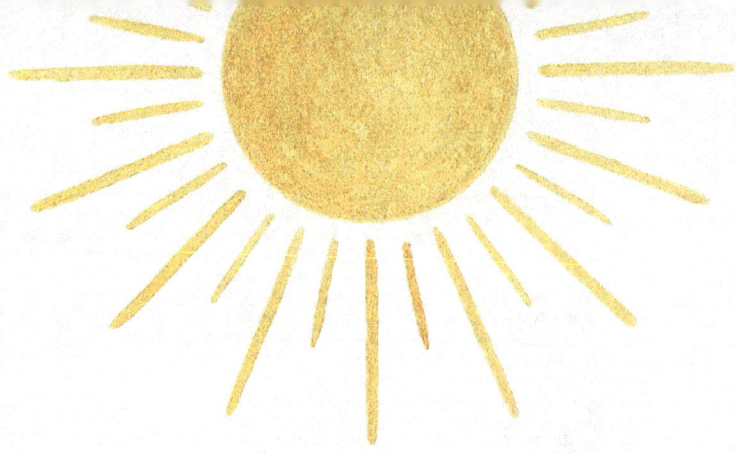

SEROTONIN — PEACE OF BALANCE AND CONTENTMENT

Vedic Principle: Sattva — Purity, Harmony, and Inner Order

Serotonin = Joy of Calm Stability.

It thrives when you cultivate simplicity, stillness, and gratitude.

Vedic Ways to Enhance Serotonin:

1. Sattvic Diet: Eat foods grown with sunlight and love — fresh fruits, ghee, milk, nuts, grains.
2. Sunlight and Surya Namaskar: Salute the sun each morning; sunlight stimulates serotonin and uplifts mood.
3. Japa (Repetition of Mantra): Soothing repetition of "Om Shanti Shanti Shantiḥ" calms the mind and stabilizes emotions.
4. Nature Walks (Prakriti Darshan): Spend time in forests, riversides, or gardens — Nature restores mental equilibrium.

Mantra for Peace: "Om Shantiḥ Antar Shantiḥ Bahir Shantiḥ Sarvatra Shantiḥ" — Peace within, peace without, peace everywhere.

OXYTOCIN — LOVE, TRUST, AND CONNECTION

Vedic Principle: Prema — Divine Love and Compassion

Oxytocin = Hormone of Bonding and Belonging.

It rises through heart-centered actions — devotion, kindness, and service.

Vedic Ways to Enhance Oxytocin:

1. Bhakti (Devotion): Sing, chant, or pray to your chosen deity with love — Krishna, Vitthala, or Sai — invoking pure connection.
2. Seva (Service): Do something selfless daily — feeding birds, helping a neighbor, caring for elders.
3. Touch & Warmth: In the Vedic family tradition, blessings and affectionate touch transmit Sneha (loving warmth).
4. Community (Satsang): Surround yourself with uplifting company; shared joy multiplies oxytocin energy.

Mantra for Love: "Prema Swaroopa Aham" — I am the embodiment of love.

ENDORPHINS — NATURAL ECSTASY AND VITAL ENERGY

Vedic Principle: Ananda Rasa — The Nectar of Joyful Flow

Endorphins = Hormones of Joy and Energy.

They arise when body and breath unite in rhythm and expression.

Vedic Ways to Enhance Endorphins:

1. Dance and Kirtan: Joyful rhythmic movement and chanting awaken blissful hormones.
2. Yoga Asanas: Especially dynamic flows like Surya Namaskar, Utkatasana, and Trikonasana stimulate vitality.
3. Laughter and Play: The Vedas celebrated joy as worship — play, laugh, express freely!
4. Aroma and Sound: Use sandalwood, rose, or lavender; listen to Vedic chants or nature sounds.

Mantra for Joy: "Anando'ham" — I am joy itself.

GABA — DEEP RELAXATION AND TRANQUILITY

Vedic Principle: Shanti — Stillness and Equanimity

GABA = Hormone of Calm and Safety.

It flows when we release control and rest in presence.

Vedic Ways to Enhance GABA:

1. Yoga Nidra (Yogic Sleep): Lie down, breathe deeply, and let go — the nervous system resets naturally.

2. Nadi Shodhana Prāṇāyāma (Alternate Nostril Breathing): Harmonizes both brain hemispheres, calming anxiety.

3. Trataka (Candle Gazing): Focus the gaze on a flame to stabilize attention and quiet the mind.

4. Night Ritual: End your day with a warm bath, chanting "Om Namo Narayanaya."

Mantra for Calm: "Shantiḥ Shantiḥ Shantiḥ" — I am peace in motion.

THE SACRED HARMONY: THE FIVE INNER ELIXIRS

Modern Hormone	Vedic Energy	Practice	Essence
Dopamine	Dharma Shakti	Purpose & Tapas	Joy of Doing
Serotonin	Sattva Guna	Meditation & Sun	Joy of Balance
Oxytocin	Prema Bhava	Bhakti & Service	Joy of Connection
Endorphins	Ananda Rasa	Yoga & Dance	Joy of Flow
GABA	Shanti Tatva	Nidra & Breath	Joy of Stillness

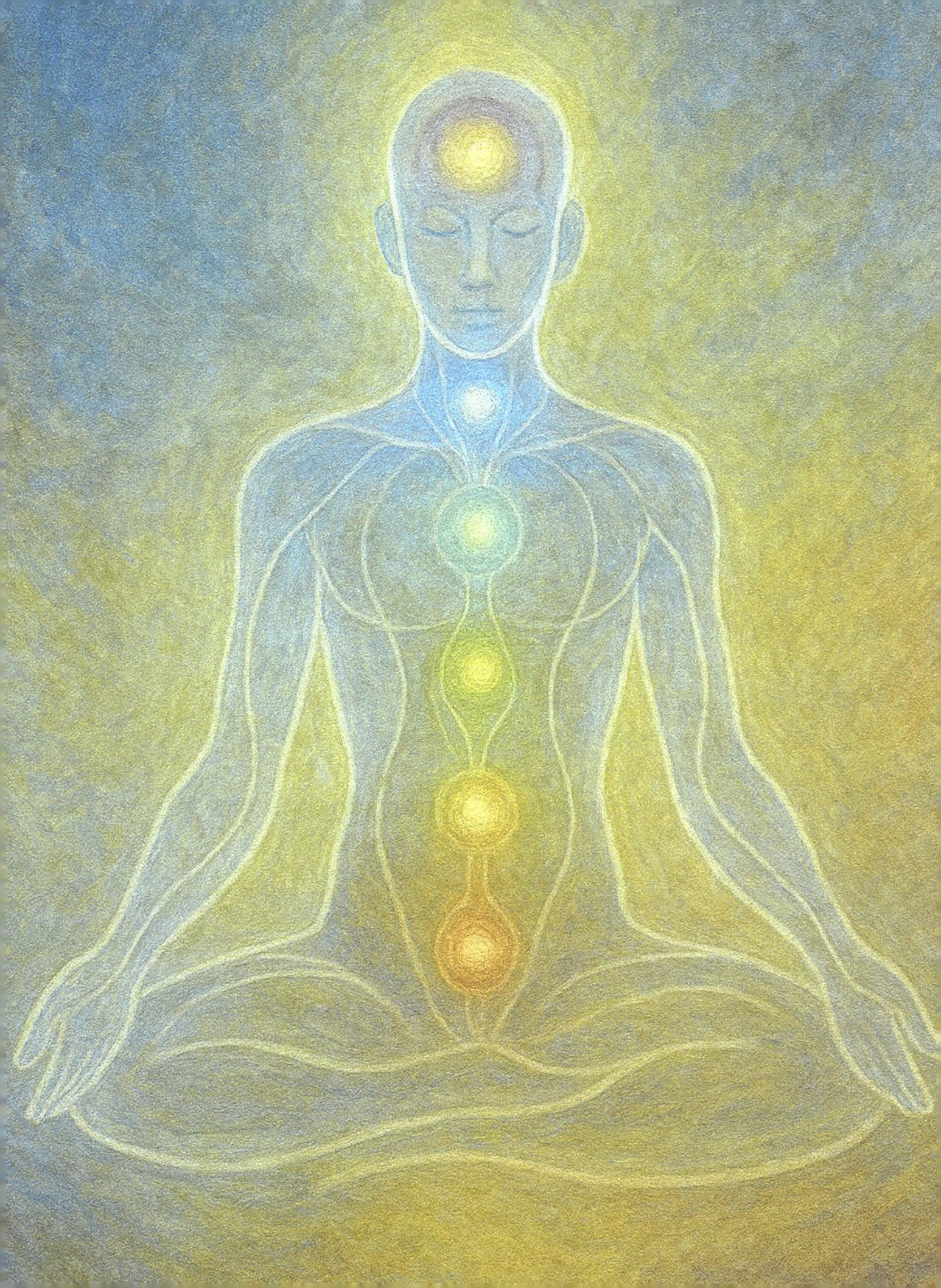

VAGAL TONE

Strengthening vagal tone means enhancing the flexibility and calm power of your parasympathetic nervous system, the "rest, digest, and heal" branch.

A well-toned vagus nerve helps regulate mood, digestion, immunity, heart rate, and emotional resilience.

Here's a complete mind–body–spirit guide to improving vagal tone, blending modern science with ancient wisdom:

1. BREATHWORK — THE GATEWAY

Slow, deep, rhythmic breathing directly stimulates the vagus nerve.
- **Technique:** Inhale for 4 counts, exhale for 6 counts.
- **Alternative:** Bhramari Pranayama (humming bee breath) — the vibration enhances vagal activity.
- **Tip:** Practice before sleep or during stress; consistency matters more than duration.

2. CHANTING, HUMMING, OR MANTRA RECITATION

The vagus nerve runs near the vocal cords — vibration and resonance stimulate it.
- **Mantras:** Om, So Hum, or any devotional mantra (Vitthala, Gayatri, etc.)
- **Duration:** 5–10 minutes of humming or chanting can reset your nervous system.
- **Bonus:** Humming before meals enhances digestion through vagal activation.

3. HEART–BRAIN COHERENCE

The heart has direct vagal connections.

- **Practice:** Focus your attention on your heart, breathe slowly, and evoke a feeling of gratitude or love.
- **Scientific benefit:** Increases heart rate variability (HRV), a measure of vagal tone.

4. COLD EXPOSURE

Gentle cold activates the vagus nerve through facial and neck pathways.

- **Simple ways:**
    - End your shower with 15–30 seconds of cool water.
    - Splash cool water on your face in the morning.
    - Breathe calmly while doing it — don't tense up.
- **Contraindication:** Avoid if you have heart or thyroid conditions without medical clearance.

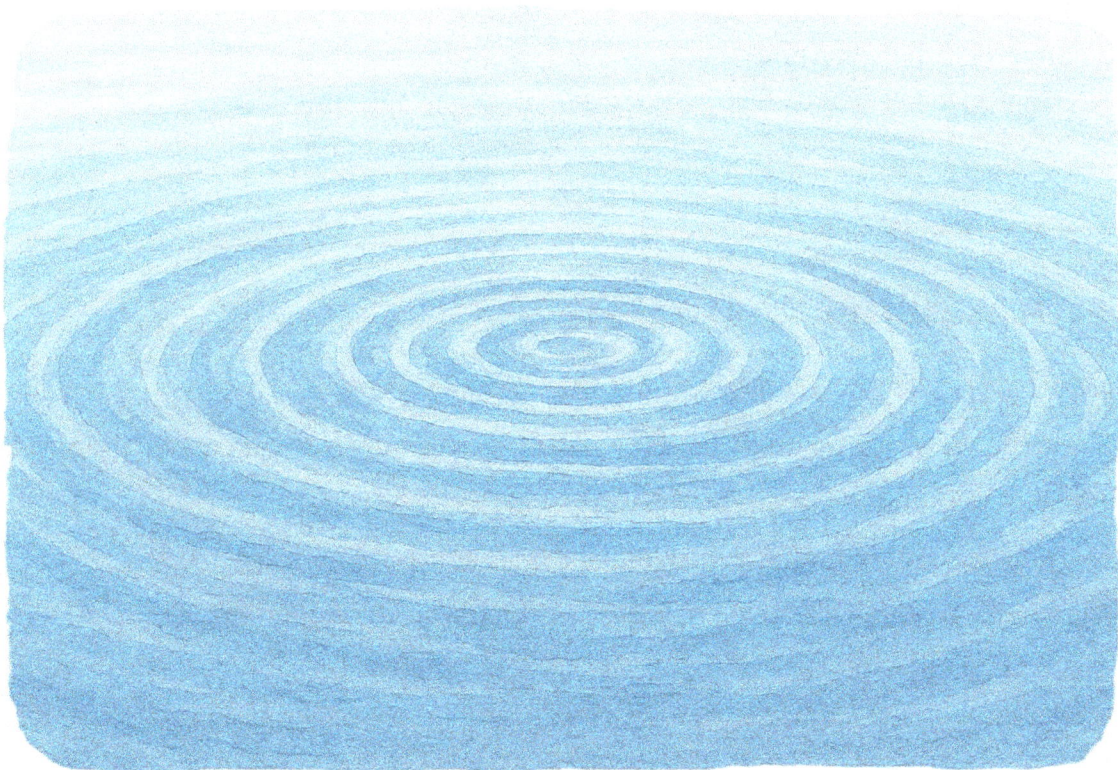

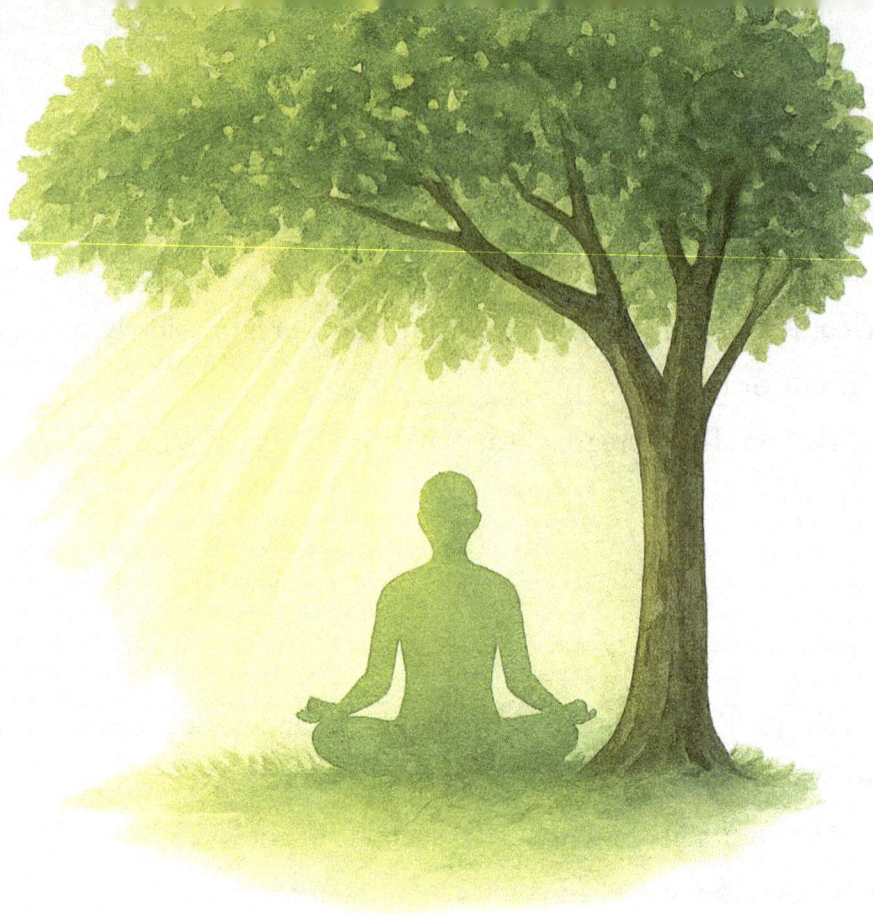

5. GROUNDING AND FOREST TIME (CHAYA CHIKITSA)

- Earthing through bare feet, forest walking, or gardening stabilizes the parasympathetic system.
- Nature's negative ions and rhythmic light exposure calm vagal circuits and balance circadian rhythm.
- Even 20 minutes of daily nature immersion works wonders.

6. GUT–BRAIN NOURISHMENT

The vagus nerve is the gut's main communicator.

- **Support with:** fermented foods (yogurt, buttermilk, sauerkraut), prebiotics (banana, garlic), and sattvic foods.
- **Avoid:** excessive stimulants, processed sugar, and inflammatory foods.
- **Ayurvedic tip:** sip warm water infused with cumin, coriander, and fennel to keep digestion gentle.

7. YOGA, MUDRA, AND POSTURE

- **Asanas:** Fish pose (Matsyasana), Camel (Ustrasana), and gentle inversions enhance vagal flow.
- **Mudra:** Chin Mudra (thumb-index connection) balances prana and promotes relaxation.
- **Restorative yoga postures:** stimulate deep relaxation responses.

8. SOUND, RHYTHM, AND LAUGHTER

- Laughter yoga boosts vagal tone through diaphragmatic movement.
- Listening to calm music or rhythmic drumming synchronizes heart and breath rhythms.
- Vedic sound therapy: use binaural beats around 432 Hz or 528 Hz with mantras for deep parasympathetic activation.

9. LOVING CONNECTION AND MINDFULNESS

The vagus nerve thrives on safety and social connection.

- Eye contact, affectionate touch, and mindful presence enhance its tone.
- Daily gratitude journaling and prayer deepen this field of calm.

10. REST AND RHYTHM

- The vagus nerve resets in predictable cycles — regular meals, sleep, and meditative pauses restore tone.
- Disorder or rushing blunts vagal responsiveness.

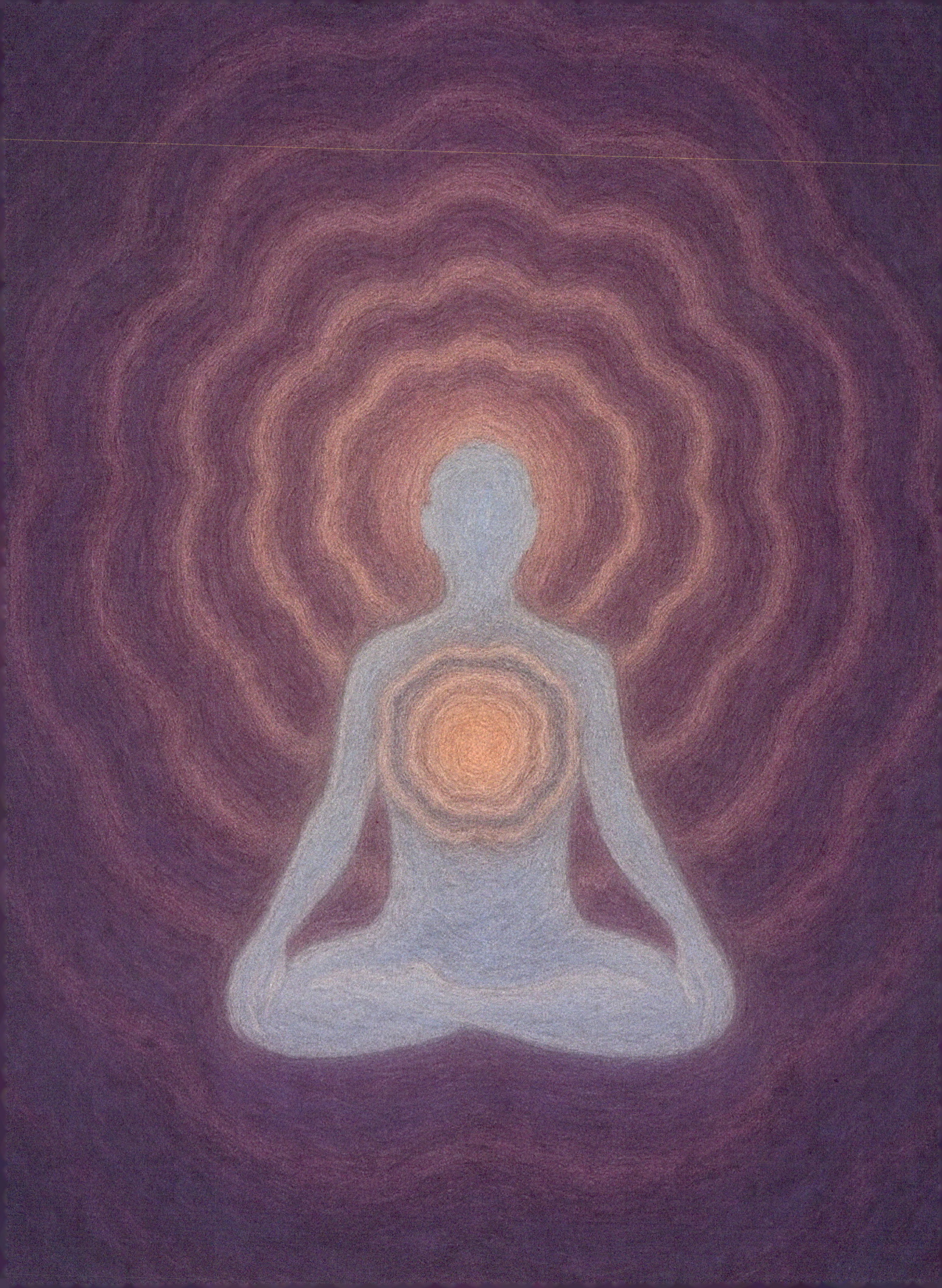

VEDIC BREATHING PRACTICES

In Vedic and Yogic science, Prāṇa (life-force) is the bridge between the body and consciousness — between the chemistry of happiness and the vibration of bliss.

When the Prāṇa flows rhythmically, the mind becomes calm, emotions settle, and hormones like serotonin, endorphins, and oxytocin are naturally balanced.

Here are 7 powerful Vedic breathing practices — simple, sacred, and science-aligned — to awaken happiness from within.

ANULOM VILOM — THE BREATH OF BALANCE (ALTERNATE NOSTRIL BREATHING)

Purpose: Harmonizes left and right brain hemispheres; stabilizes mood; enhances serotonin.

Effect: Peace, clarity, emotional stability.

How to Practice:
1. Sit comfortably with straight spine.
2. Close the right nostril with thumb, inhale slowly through the left.
3. Close the left nostril, exhale through the right.
4. Then inhale through the right, exhale through the left.
5. Continue for 7–10 cycles.

Mantra (optional): "So… Ham…" (I am That) — inhale "So", exhale "Ham."

Vedic Essence: Brings balance between Ida and Pingala — the lunar and solar energies of the mind.

BHASTRIKA PRĀṆĀYĀMA — THE BELLOWS OF JOY

Purpose: Increases energy, releases endorphins, clears emotional stagnation.

Effect: Uplifted mood, inner vitality, joyful enthusiasm.

How to Practice:

1. Sit upright, inhale deeply through both nostrils.
2. Exhale forcefully through both nostrils using abdominal muscles.
3. Repeat 10–20 times (one round). Rest.
4. Perform 3 rounds.

Mantra: "Om Hrīm Namah" — energizing mantra of light.

Vedic Essence: Awakens Agni, the inner fire of transformation, converting dullness into radiant joy.

BHRĀMARĪ PRĀṆĀYĀMA — THE HUMMING BEE BREATH

Purpose: Stimulates vagus nerve, releases oxytocin, quiets the mind.

Effect: Love, connection, calm, and emotional harmony.

How to Practice:

1. Inhale deeply.
2. Close your ears gently with thumbs.
3. Exhale slowly while humming a deep, smooth "mmm" sound.
4. Feel vibration in your head and heart.
5. Repeat 7 times.

Mantra: "Om Aim Hreem Shreem" — the feminine vibration of bliss.

Vedic Essence: Connects to the heart center (Anāhata Chakra), cultivating compassion and inner joy.

UJJĀYĪ PRĀṆĀYĀMA — THE OCEANIC BREATH OF SERENITY

Purpose: Activates parasympathetic system; increases serotonin and GABA.

Effect: Calm confidence, inner contentment, meditative state.

How to Practice:

1. Inhale through the nose while gently constricting the throat (making a whispering sound).
2. Exhale slowly with the same sound.
3. Continue for 5–7 minutes.

Mantra: "Om Shanti Shanti Shantiḥ"

Vedic Essence: Reflects the oceanic rhythm of consciousness — steady, peaceful, infinite.

KAPĀLABHĀTI — THE BREATH OF RADIANCE

Purpose: Detoxifies, energizes dopamine flow, awakens clarity.

Effect: Lightness, alert joy, mental freshness.

How to Practice:

1. Inhale normally.
2. Exhale quickly through the nose, pulling the abdomen in sharply.
3. Do 20–50 strokes, rest, then repeat 3 rounds.

Mantra: "Om Suryaaya Namaha" — invoking solar brightness.

Vedic Essence: Clears mental fog, ignites Tejas — the inner glow of awareness.

SAHAJ PRĀṆĀYĀMA — EFFORTLESS AWARENESS OF BREATH

Purpose: Deepens mindfulness; integrates all hormones of happiness.

Effect: Tranquil joy, deep rest, meditative bliss.

How to Practice:

1. Sit quietly.
2. Simply observe your natural breath — no control, no effort.
3. Feel air entering and leaving the nostrils.
4. Stay aware for 10–15 minutes.

Mantra: "Aham Brahmāsmi" — I am Divine Consciousness.

Vedic Essence: Leads to the experience of Sat-Chit-Ānanda — pure being, awareness, and bliss.

HRIDAYA PRĀṆĀYĀMA — THE BREATH OF THE HEART

Purpose: Harmonizes breath with heart rhythm; increases oxytocin and endorphins.

Effect: Emotional healing, warmth, compassion.

How to Practice:

1. Place right hand on heart.
2. Inhale to the count of 4, feeling heart expand.
3. Hold for 2 counts; exhale for 6.
4. Visualize pink-golden light radiating outward.

Mantra: "Prema Swaroopa Aham" — I am the embodiment of love.

Vedic Essence: Connects prāṇa to the heart's vibration, transforming breathing into devotion.

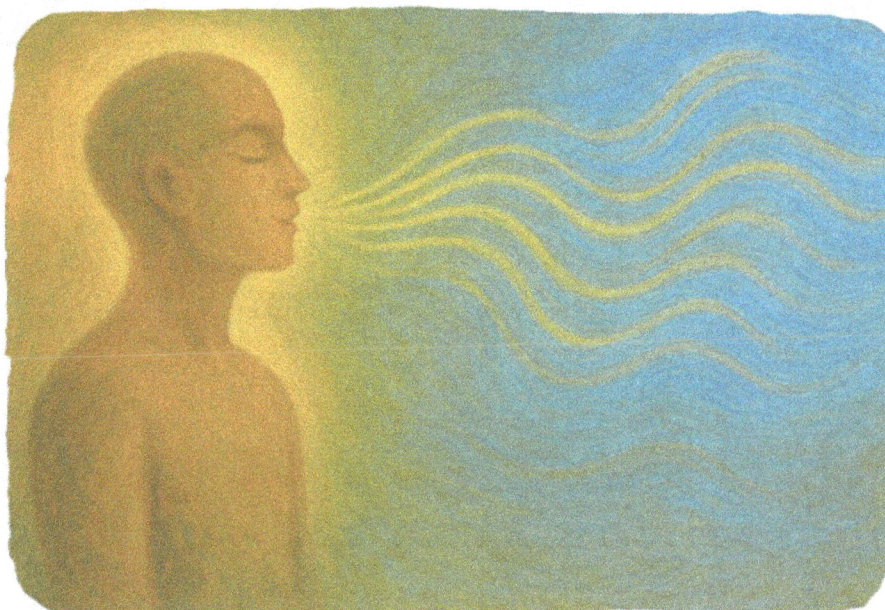

BREATHWORK ROUTINE FOR THE DAY

Time	Practice	Focus	Result
Morning	Kapālabhāti + Bhastrika	Activation	Energy, motivation
Midday	Anulom Vilom	Balance	Clarity, calm
Evening	Ujjayi + Bhramari	Relaxation	Peace, joy
Before Sleep	Hridaya or Sahaj	Stillness	Deep rest, happiness

VEDIC REFLECTION

"Breath is the silent bridge between the body and the soul.
In each conscious breath lies the doorway to bliss."
— *Vijnana Bhairava Tantra*

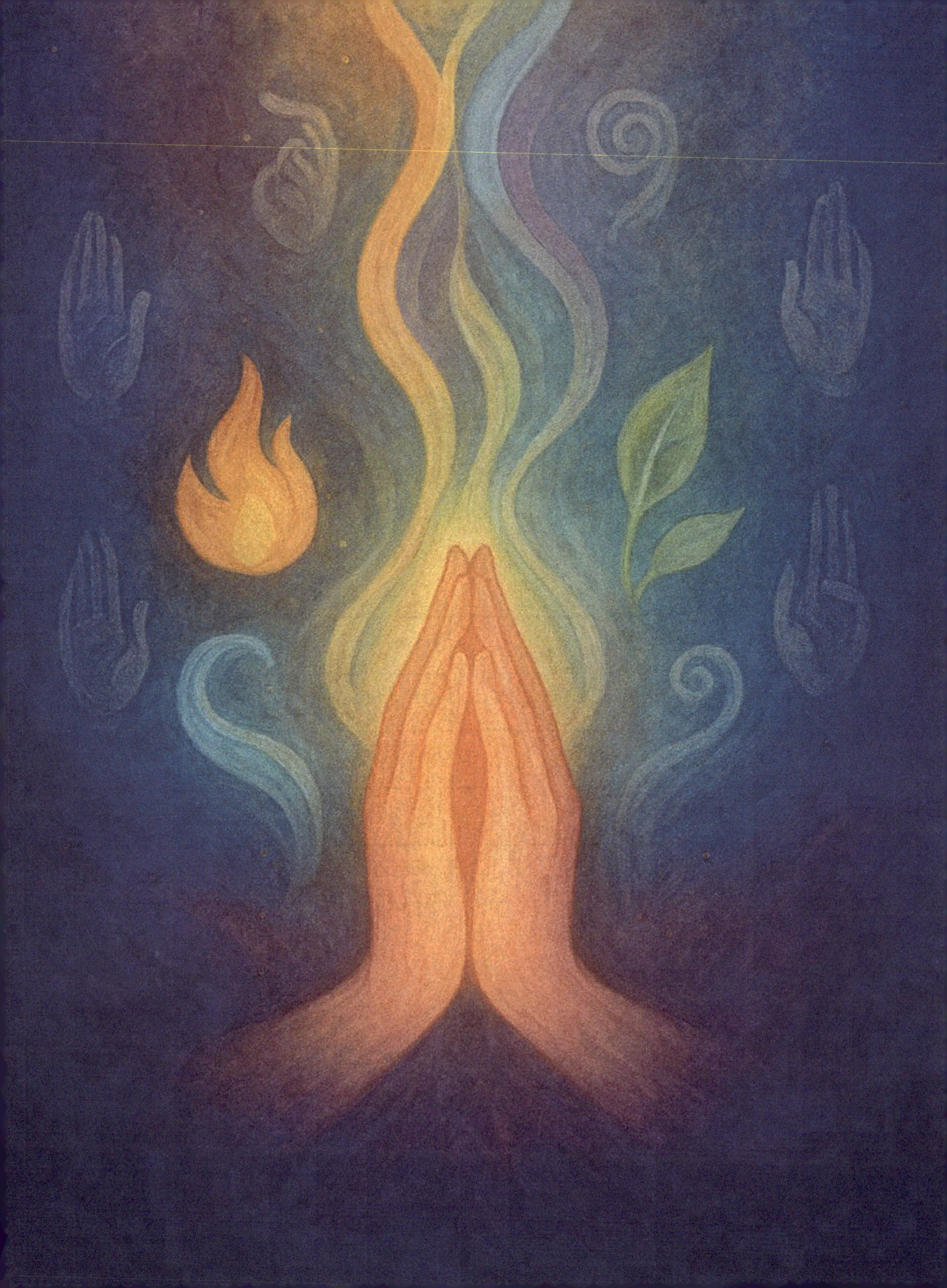

MUDRAS — THE SACRED GESTURES OF ĀNANDA

In Vedic and Yogic wisdom, Mudra (मुद्रा) literally means "seal" or "gesture." It is a divine language of the hands — where energy channels (nadis) are directed consciously to balance the five elements within. When used with breath (prāṇāyāma) and awareness (dhyāna), mudras awaken happiness hormones and harmonize the subtle body.

Below are 7 sacred mudras that open the flow of joy, peace, and inner fulfillment (Sat-Chit-Ānanda) — combining Vedic symbolism with neuro-hormonal understanding.

GYAN MUDRA — THE GESTURE OF WISDOM & CALM

Elemental Balance: Air (Vayu)

Stimulates: Serotonin, Dopamine

Activates: Brain centers of clarity, peace

Vedic Essence: Symbol of Jnana — wisdom. When the index finger (individual self) unites with the thumb (Universal Self), it dissolves ego and brings inner peace.

How to Practice:

1. Sit in Sukhasana, palms facing upward.
2. Touch the tip of thumb and index finger lightly. Keep other fingers straight.
3. Rest hands on knees. Breathe deeply for 10 minutes.

Mantra: "So'ham" — I am That.

Effect: Mental calmness, focus, serenity — awakens Sat (Truth).

PRANA MUDRA — THE GESTURE OF VITAL ENERGY

Elemental Balance: Earth + Water + Fire

Stimulates: Endorphins

Activates: Root and Heart Chakras

Vedic Essence: Known as the Life Force Seal, it activates Kundalini and enhances vitality and immunity. Brings enthusiasm and joy from within — like sunshine in the heart.

How to Practice:

1. Sit or stand comfortably.
2. Join thumb, ring finger, and little finger.
3. Practice for 15 minutes daily.

Mantra: "Om Pranaya Namaha."

Effect: Energy, optimism, radiant happiness.

HRIDAYA MUDRA — THE GESTURE OF THE HEART

Elemental Balance: Fire + Air

Stimulates: Oxytocin, Serotonin

Activates: Heart Chakra (Anāhata)

Vedic Essence: Known as Heart Gesture of Love, it releases grief and expands compassion. It opens the flow of Prema Rasa — unconditional love and acceptance.

How to Practice:

1. Bring hands to heart center.
2. Form the mudra on both hands — bring the index finger to the base of the thumb, with the thumb touching both the middle and ring fingers
3. Close eyes and inhale slowly, exhale with feeling of love.

Mantra: "Prema Swaroopa Aham."

Effect: Emotional healing, connection, and joy.

SURYA MUDRA — THE GESTURE OF INNER RADIANCE

Elemental Balance: Fire (Agni)

Stimulates: Dopamine, Endorphins

Activates: Solar Plexus (Manipura Chakra)

Vedic Essence: Represents Surya Tattva — the sun principle of vigor and clarity. It burns laziness, awakens enthusiasm, and enhances metabolism and willpower.

How to Practice:

1. Sit straight and close eyes.
2. Bend ring finger to base of thumb and press gently.
3. Practice in morning sunlight for 10 minutes.

Mantra: "Om Suryaya Namaha."

Effect: Motivation, strength, radiant happiness.

DHYANA MUDRA — THE GESTURE OF MEDITATION

Elemental Balance: Ether (Akasha)

Stimulates: Serotonin & GABA

Activates: Third Eye & Crown Chakras

Vedic Essence: Symbolizes inner stillness and unity. It is used in all Buddha and Shiva meditations. When the breath stills in this mudra, the mind merges into blissful awareness.

How to Practice:

1. Sit in Padmasana or Sukhasana.
2. Rest hands in lap, right over left, thumbs lightly touching.
3. Gaze softly inward or focus on breath.

Mantra: "Aham Brahmāsmi."

Effect: Deep peace, insight, transcendental joy.

SHAKTI MUDRA — THE GESTURE OF INNER NURTURING

Elemental Balance: Water + Earth

Stimulates: GABA, Oxytocin

Activates: Sacral Chakra (Svadhishthana)

Vedic Essence: Represents Devi Shakti, the creative, healing feminine energy. Brings deep relaxation, restful sleep, and emotional comfort.

How to Practice:

1. Place hands near navel.
2. Form the mudra — bring the tips of the ring and little fingers together on both hands, press the thumbs into the palms, and let the index and middle fingers rest over the thumbs.

Mantra: "Om Shreem Hreem Namah."

Effect: Relaxation, comfort, emotional balance.

APAN MUDRA — THE GESTURE OF EMOTIONAL RELEASE

Elemental Balance: Fire + Space + Earth

Stimulates: Detox hormones & serotonin

Activates: Solar & Root Chakras

Vedic Essence: Known as Mudra of Letting Go, it aids in emotional purification. When inner blockages dissolve, bliss arises naturally.

How to Practice:

1. Sit comfortably with eyes closed.
2. Touch thumb to middle and ring fingers
3. Hold the mudra for 10 minutes while breathing deeply.

Mantra: "Om Apanaya Namaha."

Effect: Detoxification, release, inner freedom.

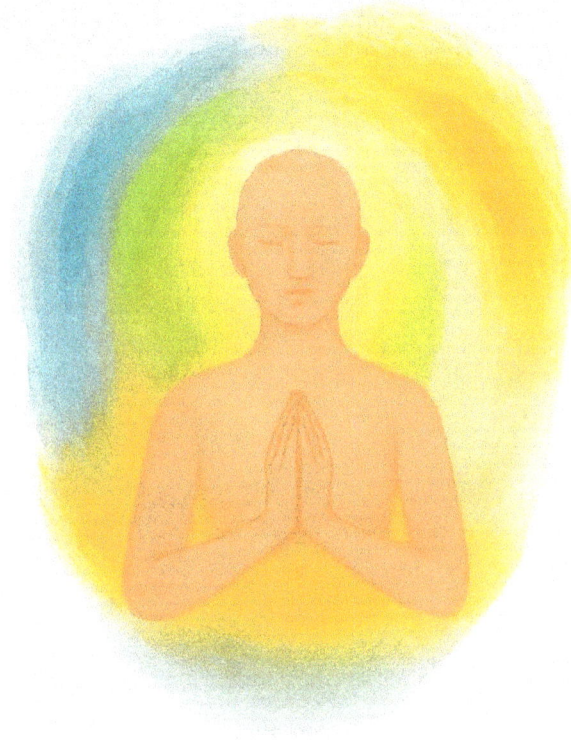

MUDRA ROUTINE FOR THE DAY

Time	Mudra	Essence	Result
Morning	Surya + Prana	Energy, activation	Joyful motivation
Midday	Gyan	Focus, clarity	Calm awareness
Evening	Hridaya + Shakti	Love, nurturing	Emotional harmony
Before Sleep	Dhyana	Stillness	Deep peace & bliss

VEDIC REFLECTION

Through each gesture of awareness, the five elements return to harmony,
and the Self shines as Ānanda — bliss without cause.

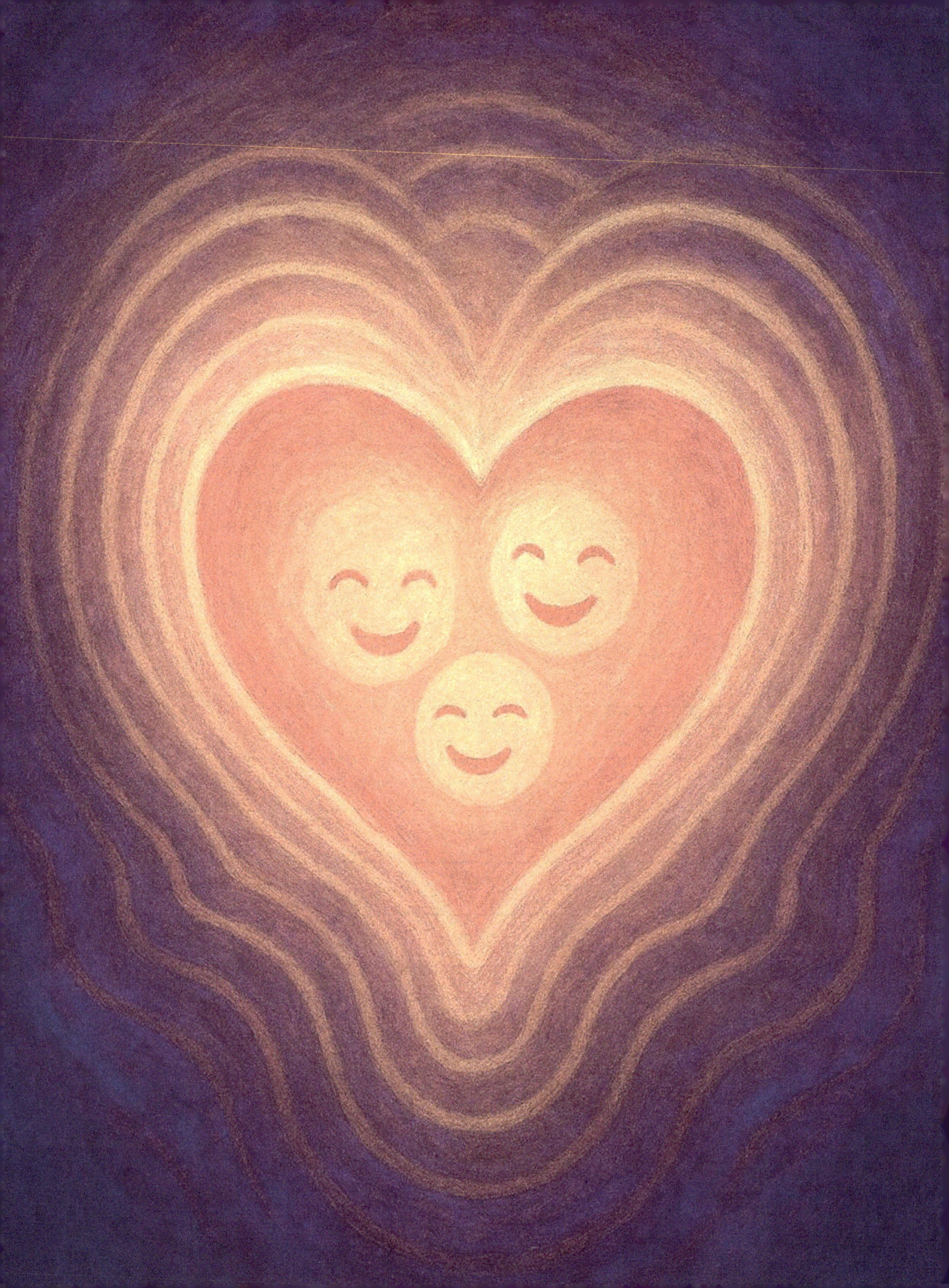

HASYA YOGA — THE YOGA OF JOYFUL LAUGHTER

Hasya Yoga (Laughter Yoga) — also known as the Yoga of Joyful Laughter — is a practice rooted in both ancient Vedic wisdom and modern yogic psychology.

Here's a concise overview from the Vedic and energetic perspective:

MEANING AND ORIGIN

- The word Hasya (हास्य) means laughter or joyful expression in Sanskrit.
- In the Nāṭya Śāstra, Hasya is one of the Navarasa — the nine sacred emotional essences. It represents lightness of being, cheerfulness, and purification of the heart.
- From the yogic viewpoint, Hasya is seen as a form of prāṇa expansion — laughter releases blocked energy and enhances ojas (vital radiance).

SPIRITUAL ESSENCE

In the Vedas, joy (ānanda) is the foundation of creation. Taittirīya Upaniṣad says: "Ānando brahmeti vyajānāt" — Bliss is Brahman.

Through laughter, we reconnect with this Ānanda-tattva, our natural state of happiness beyond intellect or ego.

ENERGETIC AND HEALTH BENEFITS

- Activates Sahasrāra (Crown Chakra) and Anāhata (Heart Chakra)
- Balances the Vāta dosha (air element), which governs nervous system and mood
- Boosts oxygenation, improves circulation, and releases endorphins
- Clears emotional stagnation and resets the mind-body rhythm

PRACTICE

1. Start with breath: Inhale deeply through the nose, exhale with a soft "haaa" sound.
2. Smile consciously: Bring awareness to the lips and eyes, inviting lightness.
3. Begin gentle laughter: Even if it feels "pretend," the body responds as real.
4. Group resonance: When done together, laughter becomes nāda (sacred sound), harmonizing subtle bodies.
5. End with silence: Feel the afterglow — the ānanda śakti spreading through the heart.

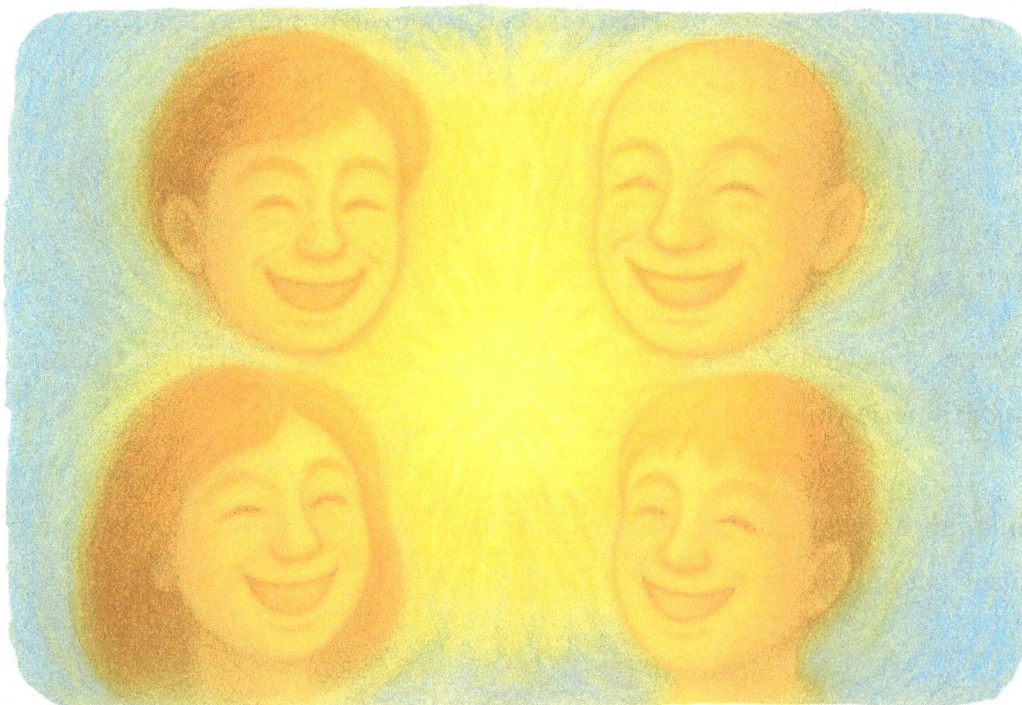

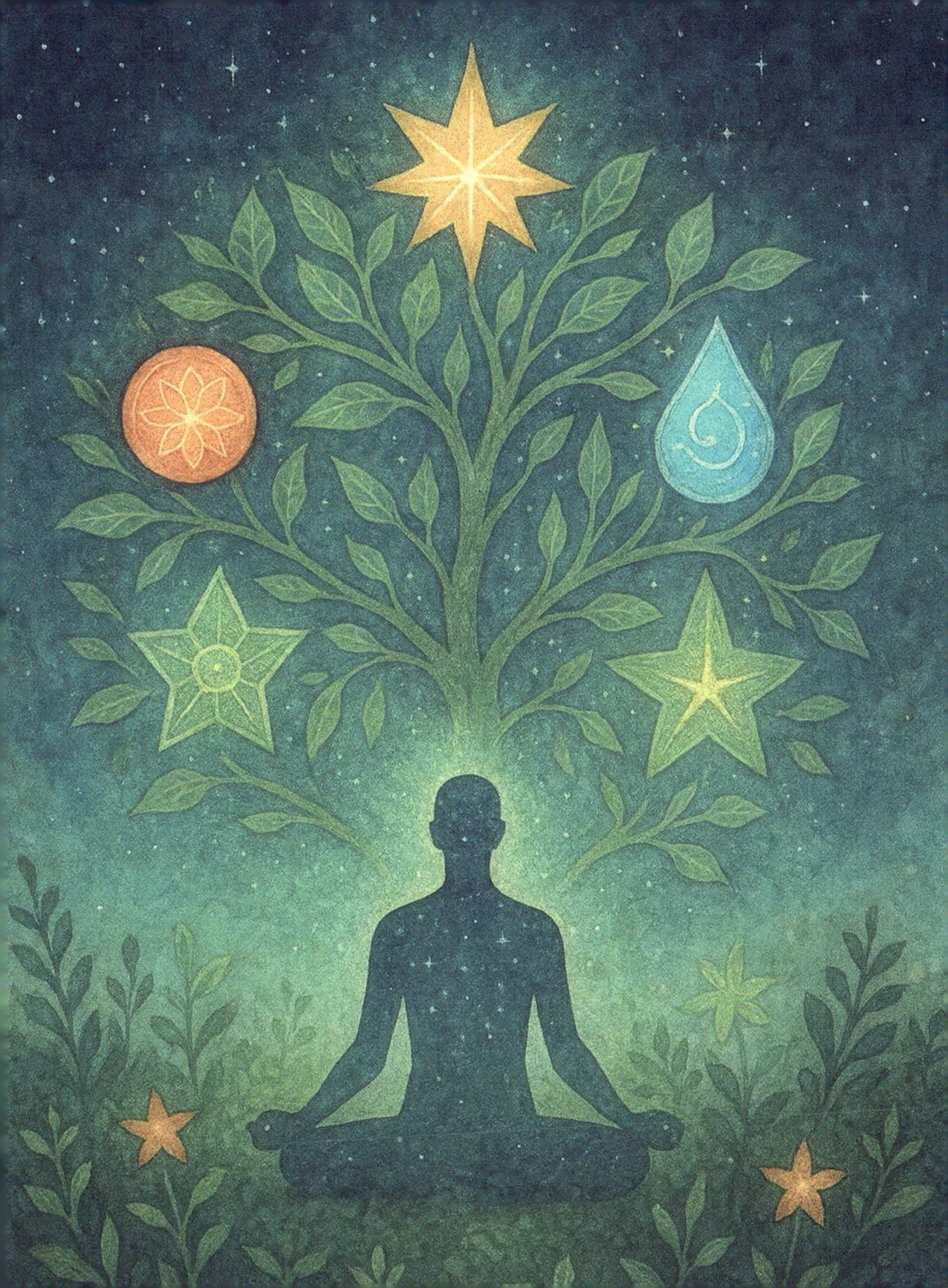

CHAYA CHIKITSA & FOREST THERAPY

THE ESSENCE

Chaya (shadow or shade) in Sanskrit signifies the cool, reflective aspect of light — the zone where intensity softens and balance returns.

When we rest under trees, walk through filtered sunlight, or sit near the forest edge, our bioelectrical field synchronizes with Earth's calm frequency (~7.83 Hz) — the Schumann resonance.

This is not symbolic alone — it:
- Reduces cortisol and blood pressure
- Enhances vagal tone
- Promotes alpha brain waves (serenity and flow)
- Revives ojas — the subtle essence of joy and immunity

"Where sunlight becomes soft and silence becomes sound — there begins healing."

VEDIC PSYCHOLOGY OF THE FOREST

In Vedic thought, the Aranya (forest) is not wilderness, but the mind's mirror. When we enter it in silence, nature begins to read our aura. Unlike human diagnostics that label, the forest senses our imbalance through vibration — and heals by subtle resonance. Each tree emits phytochemicals (phytoncides) that calm the limbic system, restore breathing rhythm, and open the heart chakra.

Element	Forest Expression	Inner Effect	Associated Hormone / Neurochemical
Air (Vayu)	Gentle wind, rustling leaves	Lightness, flow	Dopamine
Water (Jala)	Flowing streams, dew	Emotional clarity	Serotonin
Fire (Agni)	Filtered sunlight	Purpose, warmth	Endorphins
Earth (Prithvi)	Soil, roots, bark	Groundedness	Oxytocin
Ether (Akasha)	Birdsong, space between trees	Stillness, awe	GABA + melatonin

THE FOREST HAPPINESS RITUAL (CHAYA SADHANA)

MORNING: ENTERING THE GREEN SILENCE (10–15 MIN)

- Walk slowly under trees, without phone or talk.
- Match your breath to the rhythm of the rustling leaves — slow inhale, slower exhale.
- Touch a tree or sit beneath one; feel its cool shade.
- Whisper inwardly: "Let your calm become mine." This harmonizes the vagus nerve through sensory stillness and heart–earth coherence.

MIDDAY: GROUNDING PAUSE

- Sit in dappled sunlight or under shade.
- Gaze at the interplay of light and shadow on the leaves.
- Notice how joy emerges not from brightness, but from balance.
- This subtle awareness builds Santosha — contentment born of moderation.

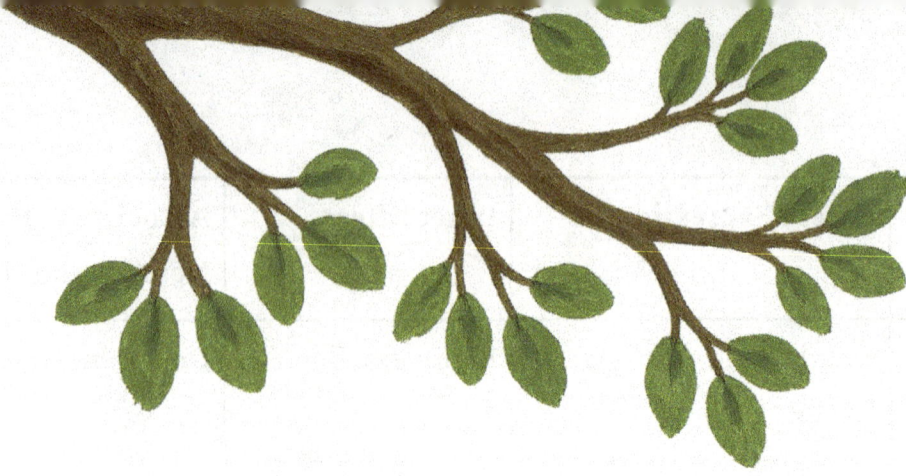

EVENING: FOREST GRATITUDE MEDITATION (10 MIN)

- Sit or visualize yourself in a forest bathed in twilight glow.

- Place hands on heart and say: "The trees breathe for me, I breathe for them."

- Imagine green light descending through your crown to your heart, then roots growing from your feet into the soil.

- End with mantra: "Om Shanti Vanadevate Namah" (Salutations to the Goddess of the Forest and Peace.)

AYURVEDIC INTEGRATION

- After forest time, drink herbal tea of tulsi, brahmi, or lemongrass — they extend the forest's calming vibration into your body.

- Light dhoop of sandalwood or vetiver in the evening — it recreates forest prana indoors.

- Apply a drop of lotus or rose oil on your heart chakra to hold the mood of peace.

REFLECTION: CHAYA AS INNER SHADE

Sometimes happiness does not come from adding more light, but from finding the sacred shade within. Chaya Chikitsa teaches that shade is not the absence of light — it is the gentleness of light. In that balance, the mind cools, hormones harmonize, and joy naturally arises.

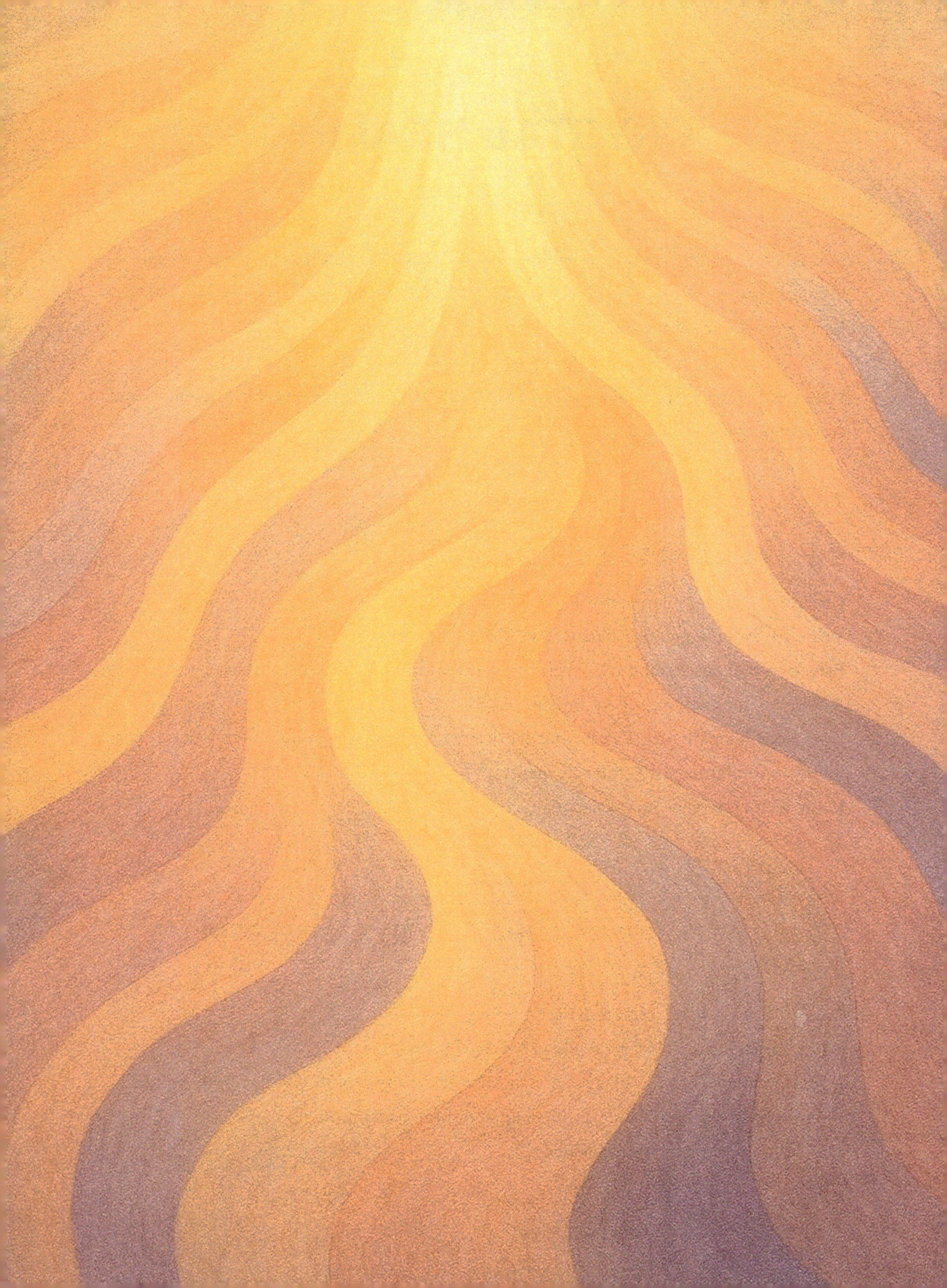

CRYSTAL HEALING

Crystals are powerful tools to enhance vagal tone, happiness, and inner steadiness because they regulate subtle vibrations in the body's energy field and synchronize with Earth's magnetic resonance.

Here's a Vedic-Energetic map of how to use crystals for happiness, blending emotional, elemental, and vagal wisdom:

CITRINE – THE SUN STONE

Energy: Uplifting, solar, joyful

Vedic Element: Agni (fire) balanced by Tejas of the heart

Effect: Stimulates serotonin and activates the Manipura (solar plexus) chakra — boosting self-worth, motivation, and optimism.

Use: Keep a small citrine near your work area or wear as a pendant; energize it with morning sunlight and a "gratitude mantra."

Mantra: "Om Hreem Suryaya Namah"

GREEN AVENTURINE – THE STONE OF CHEERFUL FLOW

Energy: Gentle, heart-centered, harmonizing

Vedic Element: Prithvi (earth) with a touch of Vayu (air)

Effect: Activates heart coherence and vagal calm; invites emotional flexibility and luck.

Use: Place on the heart while doing deep breathing or humming.

Mantra: "Om Shanti Hridaya Namah"

AQUAMARINE – THE OCEAN OF EASE

Energy: Cooling, clarifying, flowing

Vedic Element: Jala (water)

Effect: Calms anxiety and helps release emotional rigidity; tones the vagus nerve through the throat center (Vishuddha Chakra).

Use: Hold during chanting or pranayama; perfect for evening wind-down.

Mantra: "Om Vam Vishuddhaya Namah"

ROSE QUARTZ – THE HEART RESTORER

Energy: Compassionate, nurturing

Vedic Element: Soma (moon nectar)

Effect: Deepens love, forgiveness, and emotional warmth — all vagal enhancers.

Use: Keep under your pillow or in your meditation altar.

Mantra: "Om Chandraya Namah"

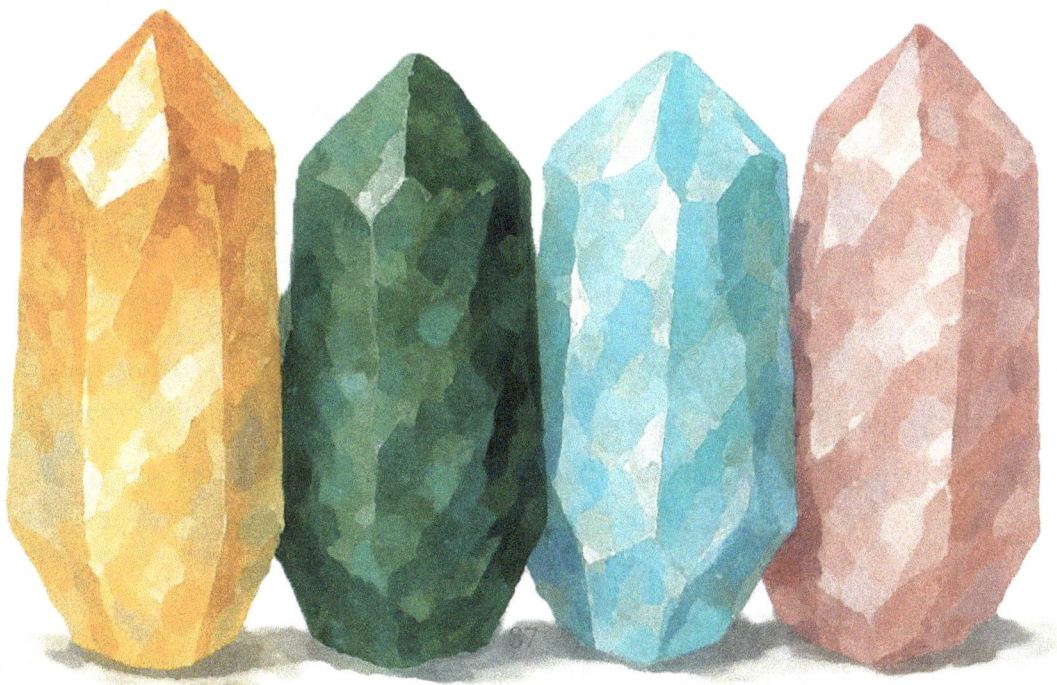

SMOKY QUARTZ – THE GROUNDING STONE

Energy: Stabilizing, detoxifying

Vedic Element: Bhumi (earth)

Effect: Anchors energy, relieves overthinking, and supports root–vagus connection.

Use: Hold while walking barefoot outdoors or during forest visualization (Chaya Chikitsa).

Mantra: "Om Prithvaye Namah"

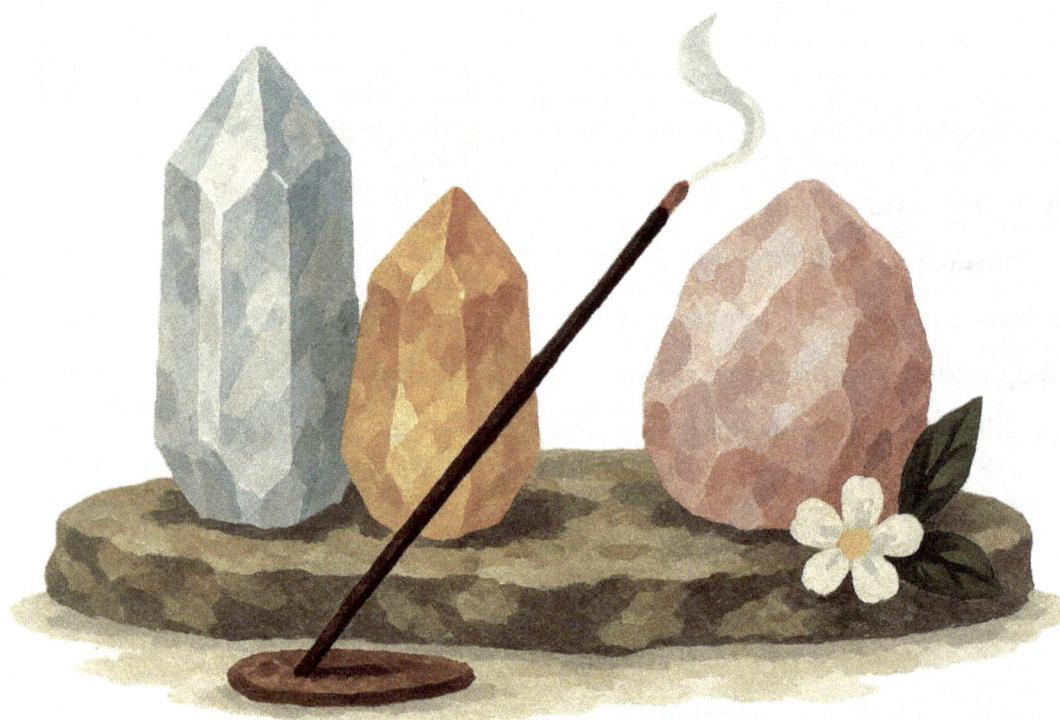

CRYSTAL + GROUNDING SYNERGY

- **Morning:** Citrine in sunlight, grounding breath, gratitude.
- **Midday:** Aventurine for emotional flow and laughter.
- **Evening:** Rose Quartz or Smoky Quartz while barefoot or meditating.
- **Weekly ritual:** Rinse crystals in running water or moonlight, offer incense or flowers as gratitude.

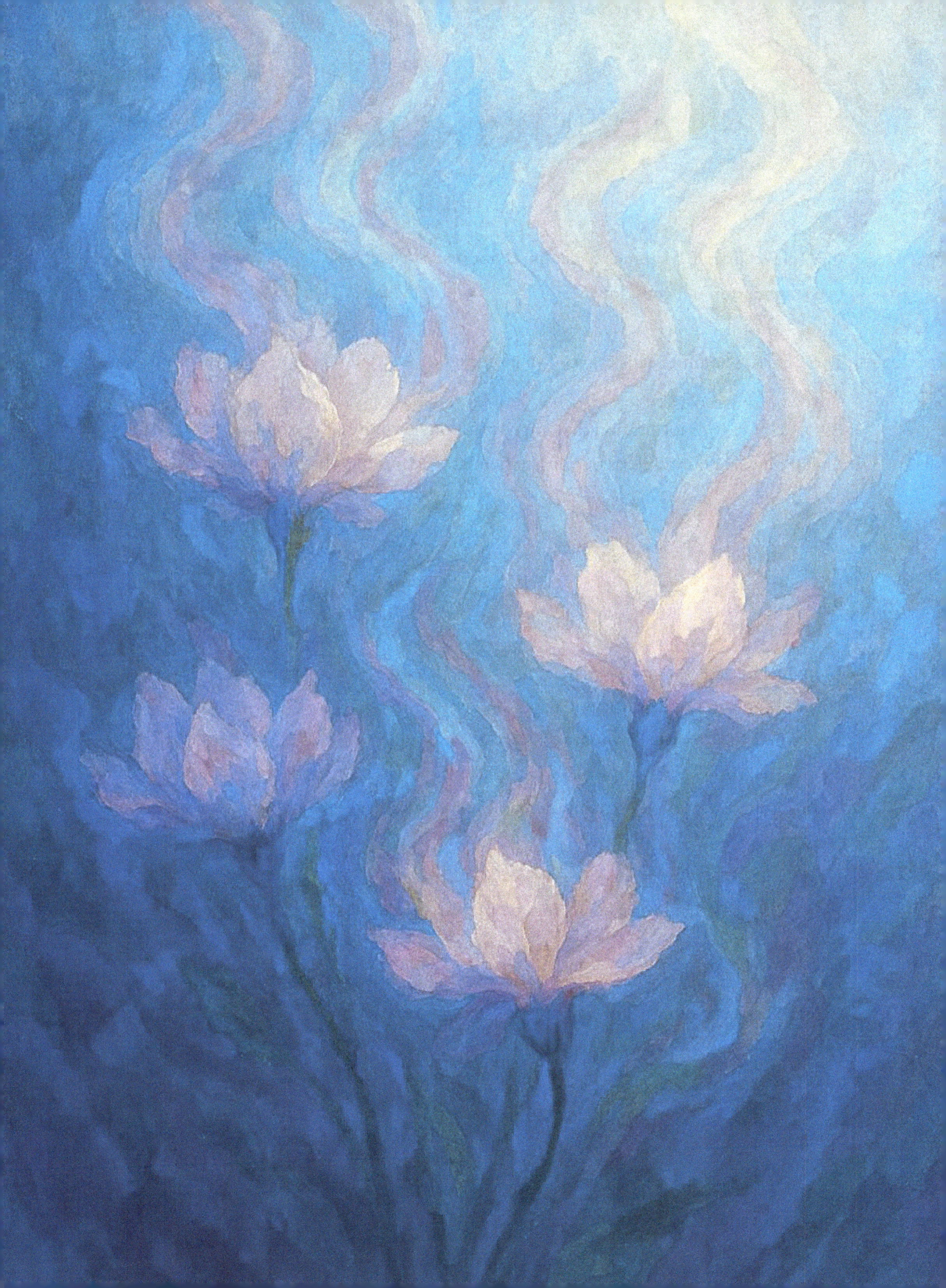

AROMATHERAPY

In Vedic tradition, fragrance (Gandha) is not just sensual pleasure — it is a subtle bridge between matter and consciousness.

The Charaka Samhita calls aroma "Manonugraha" — "that which uplifts the mind."

Each scent carries a vibration that aligns with one or more of the five elements (Pancha Mahabhutas) and influences our inner chemistry — our happiness hormones.

SANDALWOOD (CHANDANA) — PEACE, STABILITY, AND INNER JOY

Element: Earth + Water

Dosha Balance: Calms Pitta and Vata

Hormonal Resonance: Serotonin & GABA

Vedic Insight: Sandalwood is Sattva-pradhana — it stabilizes emotions and quiets restlessness. It was used in meditation and temple rituals to maintain inner coolness and peace.

Use:

- Diffuse sandalwood oil during meditation or prayer.
- Apply a small dot to the heart or Ajna chakra with coconut oil.

Recite: "Om Shanti Shanti Shantiḥ" as the aroma fills the space.

Effect: Deep tranquility, lowered anxiety, and uplifted serenity.

ROSE (SHATAPATRI) — LOVE, COMPASSION, AND HEART AWAKENING

Element: Water + Air

Dosha Balance: Balances Pitta

Hormonal Resonance: Oxytocin

Vedic Insight: Rose is the flower of Bhakti — it expands the heart and brings gentleness. In Ayurveda, rose water is used to pacify emotional heat and enhance Prema Bhava (feeling of love).

Use:

- Mist rose water on your face or pillow before meditation or rest.
- Diffuse rose oil while doing metta (loving-kindness) meditation.

Chant: "Prema Swaroopa Aham" — I am the embodiment of love.

Effect: Emotional healing, self-love, connection, and open-hearted joy.

FRANKINCENSE (LOBAN / DHOOP) — CLARITY, REVERENCE, AND SPIRITUAL UPLIFTMENT

Element: Ether + Fire

Dosha Balance: Reduces Kapha and Vata

Hormonal Resonance: Dopamine

Vedic Insight: Burned during yajñas and prayers, frankincense purifies spaces and awakens devotion. Its aroma enhances alertness while calming mental fog, bringing purpose and reverence.

Use:

- Burn a small amount as incense during sunrise meditation or chanting.
- Inhale gently to clear mental clutter before creative work.

Affirm: "Om Tat Sat" — I act in truth and awareness.

Effect: Focus, motivation, spiritual clarity, and centered enthusiasm.

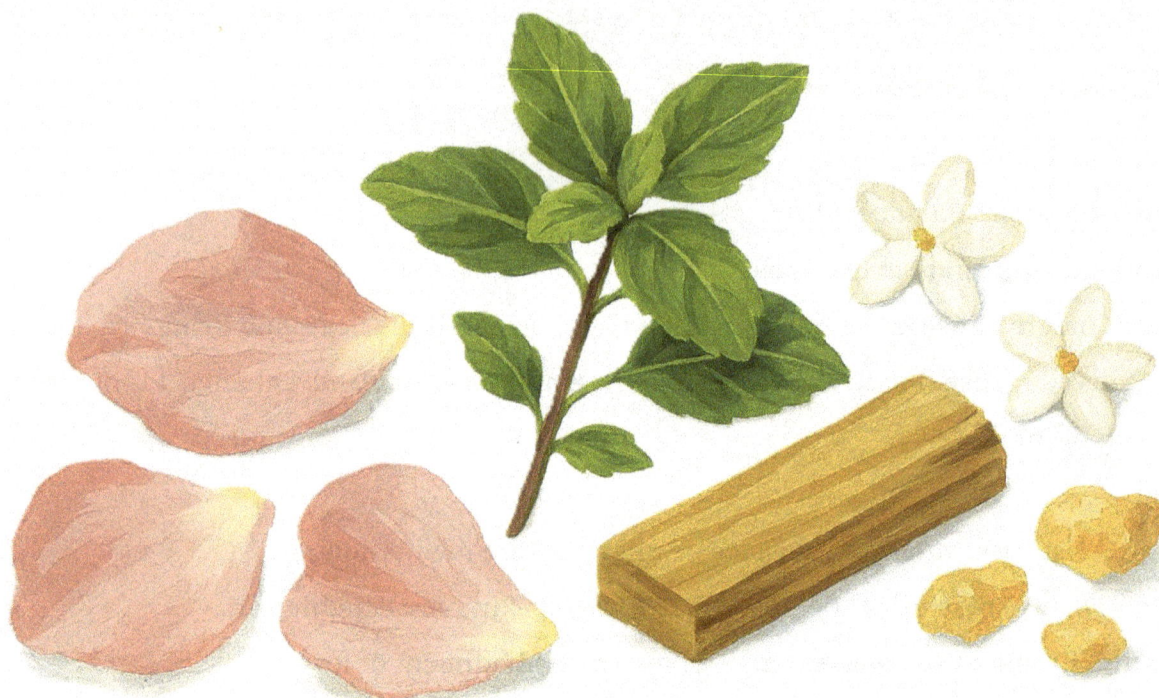

TULSI (HOLY BASIL) — VITALITY, DEVOTION, AND DIVINE PROTECTION

Element: Fire + Air

Dosha Balance: Balances Kapha and Vata

Hormonal Resonance: Endorphins & Dopamine

Vedic Insight: Tulsi is considered a living goddess — Devi Tulasi. Her fragrance energizes prana, opens the lungs, and awakens devotion (Bhakti).

Use:

- Diffuse Tulsi oil in your morning yoga or chanting practice.
- Drink Tulsi tea to enhance clarity and uplift mood.

Chant: "Om Namo Bhagavate Vasudevaya."

Effect: Energizing joy, devotion, and immunity-enhanced vitality.

JASMINE (MALLIKA) — ELATION, SENSUAL JOY, AND CREATIVE FLOW

Element: Water + Fire

Dosha Balance: Balances Vata

Hormonal Resonance: Endorphins & Oxytocin

Vedic Insight: Jasmine was used in night rituals and offered to deities of love (like Krishna and Rukmini). It relaxes the nervous system, inspires poetry and art, and stirs the inner rasa of joy.

Use:

- Diffuse jasmine oil in evening relaxation or chanting.
- Add 1-2 drops to your bath before full moon meditation.

Affirm: "Anando'ham" — I am the fragrance of bliss itself.

Effect: Euphoria, creativity, sensual balance, divine feminine energy.

VETIVER (KHUS) — GROUNDING, COOLING, AND DEEP CONTENTMENT

Element: Earth

Dosha Balance: Reduces Vata and Pitta

Hormonal Resonance: Serotonin

Vedic Insight: Vetiver roots were placed in drinking water to cool and purify it. Known as "Oil of Tranquility", it anchors wandering thoughts and provides deep rest.

Use:

- Diffuse before sleep or apply diluted to soles of feet.
- Perfect after yoga nidra or pranayama.

Chant: "Om Prithvi Devyai Namaha" — honoring Mother Earth.

Effect: Emotional grounding, restful sleep, and quiet happiness.

LEMONGRASS OR SWEET ORANGE — POSITIVITY AND FRESH ENERGY

Element: Air + Fire

Dosha Balance: Reduces Kapha

Hormonal Resonance: Dopamine & Endorphins

Vedic Insight: Citrus oils awaken Utsaha (enthusiasm) and dispel tamas (lethargy). They correspond to the solar energy of Surya, infusing brightness and renewal.

Use:

- Diffuse in workspace or during morning ritual.
- Combine with sandalwood for balanced upliftment.

Chant: "Om Suryaya Namaha."

Effect: Cheerfulness, motivation, and light-hearted creativity.

LOTUS — HAPPINESS & DIVINE BLISS (ĀNANDA DRAVYA)

Element: Water + Ether

Dosha Balance: Reduces Pitta and Vata

Hormonal Resonance: Serotonin & Oxytocin

Vedic Insight: The sacred Padma (Lotus) embodies purity rising above chaos — the awakening of the Ānandamaya Kosha, the sheath of bliss. Associated with Lakshmi (abundance) and Saraswati (wisdom), its fragrance harmonizes heart and mind, invoking serenity and inner radiance.

Use:

- Anoint the heart (Anāhata) and brow (Ājñā) centers before meditation.
- Blend with sesame or coconut oil for a heart-soothing massage.

Chant: "Om Padma Priyaye Namaha."

Effect: Opens the heart to unconditional love, serenity, and blissful awareness — radiant, serene, and ever-joyful within.

VEDIC AROMATHERAPY RITUAL FOR HAPPINESS (MORNING PRACTICE)

1. Begin with 3 deep breaths.

2. Light a diya (lamp) and say mentally: "May this fragrance purify my mind and open my heart to bliss."

3. Diffuse sandalwood or tulsi oil for grounding.

4. Add rose or jasmine for heart activation.

5. Sit in stillness for 7 minutes, letting breath and aroma merge.

6. End with "Om Anandam Brahman" — "Bliss is the essence of my being."

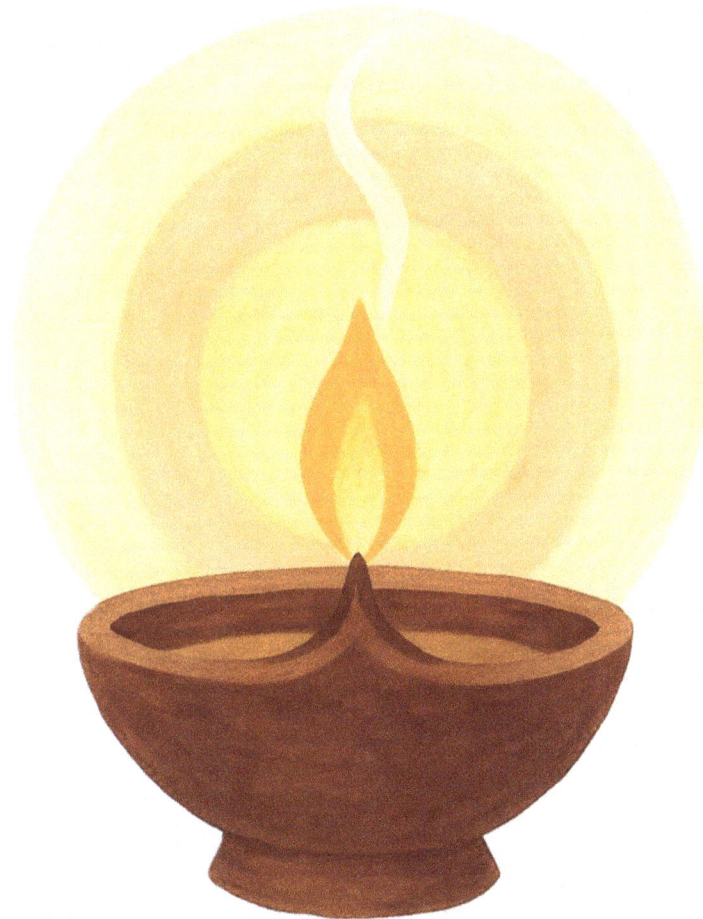

VEDIC AROMAS & HAPPINESS HORMONES

Aroma	Vedic Energy	Hormone	Effect	Mantra
Sandalwood	Shanti (Peace)	Serotonin	Calm, clarity	Om Shantiḥ
Rose	Prema (Love)	Oxytocin	Compassion	Prema Swaroopa Aham
Frankincense	Tapas (Purpose)	Dopamine	Focus, devotion	Om Tat Sat
Tulsi	Bhakti (Vitality)	Endorphins	Joy, purity	Om Namo Bhagavate
Jasmine	Rasa (Delight)	Oxytocin & Endorphins	Creativity	Anando'ham
Vetiver	Prithvi (Grounding)	Serotonin	Stability	Om Prithvi Devyai
Lemongrass	Surya (Radiance)	Dopamine	Positivity	Om Suryaya Namaha
Lotus	Ānanda (Divine Bliss)	Serotonin & Oxytocin	Serenity,	Om Padma Priyaye Namaha

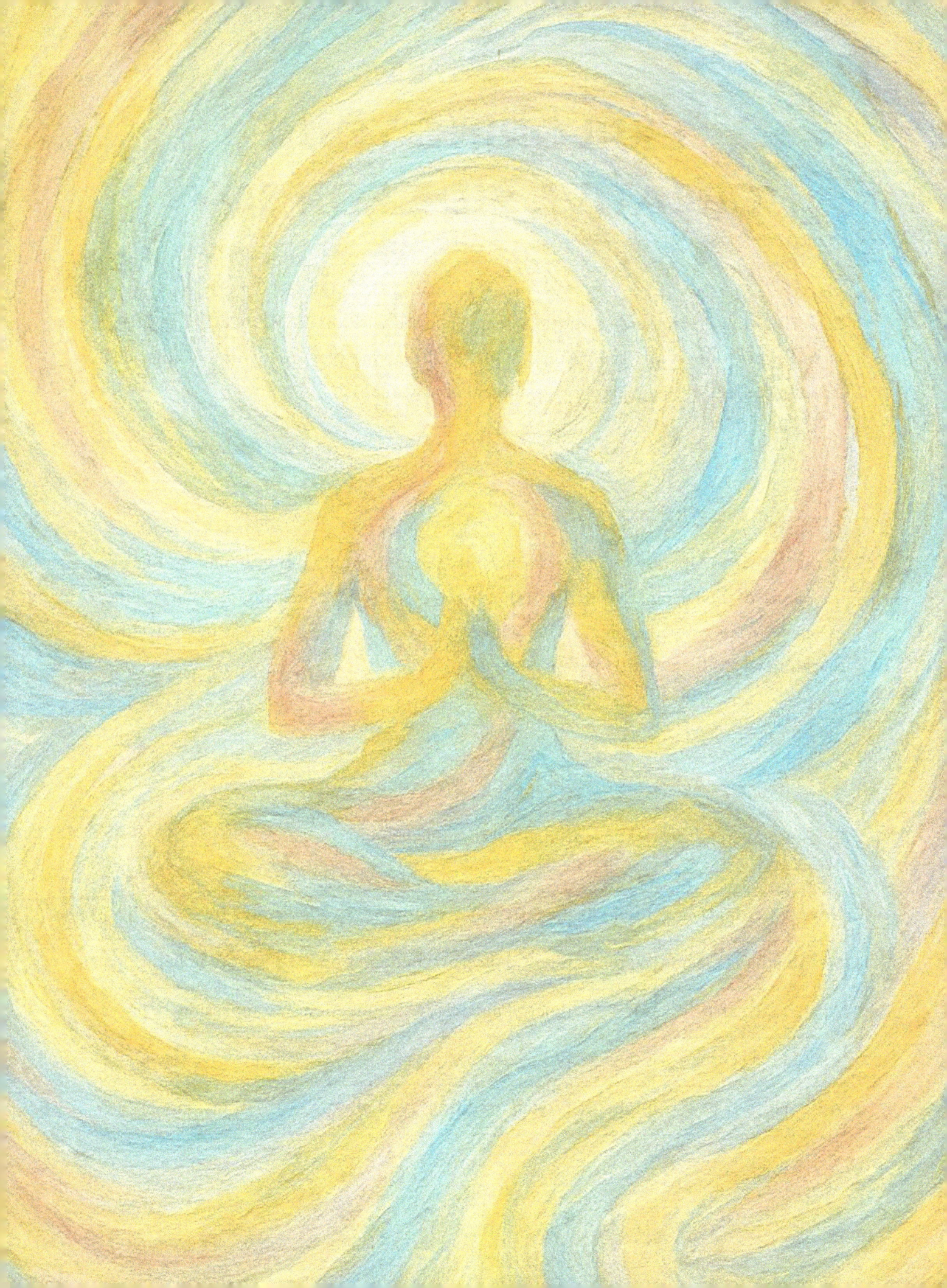

EXPLORING YOUR CREATIVE SIDE FOR JOY

Exploring your creative side for joy" is deeply aligned with the Vedic view of happiness as self-expression of the soul (Ātman's lila — the divine play). Let's unfold this idea through the lens of Vedic psychology and energy awareness:

THE SOURCE OF JOY

In the Taittirīya Upaniṣad, the seers proclaim: "Ānando brahma iti vyajānāt" — Bliss is the nature of the Divine. Creativity, in this sense, is the soul's remembrance of its divine essence. When we paint, sing, write, dance, or dream, we are not creating — we are revealing what already exists within consciousness.

THE ENERGETIC MEANING OF CREATIVITY

Every act of creation awakens certain chakras and elements:

Energy Center	Element	Creative Expression	Inner Joy
Swadhisthana (Sacral)	Water	Flow, dance, art, imagination	Pleasure in being
Anahata (Heart)	Air	Poetry, music, love, connection	Compassionate joy
Vishuddha (Throat)	Ether	Voice, truth, storytelling	Expressive freedom
Ajna (Third Eye)	Light	Vision, intuition, symbolic art	Joy of insight

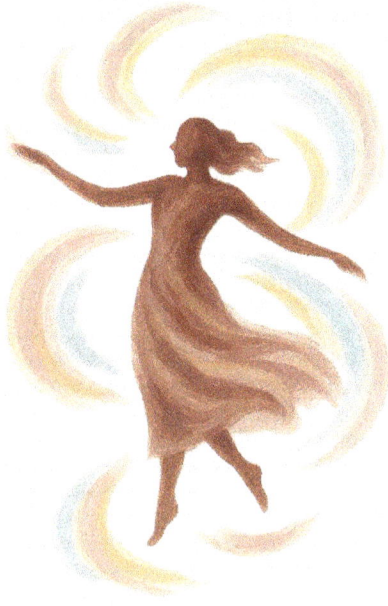

CREATIVE JOY AS SĀDHANĀ (SPIRITUAL PRACTICE)

Try these gentle practices:

- Morning Offering: Before creating, close your eyes and say — "May this act be an offering to the Divine within me."
- Color Meditation: Let each color you use represent a feeling — not a form. This bypasses the mind and lets prāṇa express through you.
- Sonic Flow: Hum softly while creating — it awakens Vishuddha and quiets self-judgment.
- Gratitude Pause: When finished, sit in silence for a moment. Notice the joy — not from completion, but from connection.

THE VEDIC UNDERSTANDING OF JOYFUL CREATION

"Sṛṣṭi hi Ānanda lakṣaṇā" — Creation itself is the mark of joy.

Just as the universe was born from Brahman's delight, your creativity is a microcosm of that same blissful expansion. True joy comes not from perfecting art, but from participating in this cosmic dance — the Līlā.

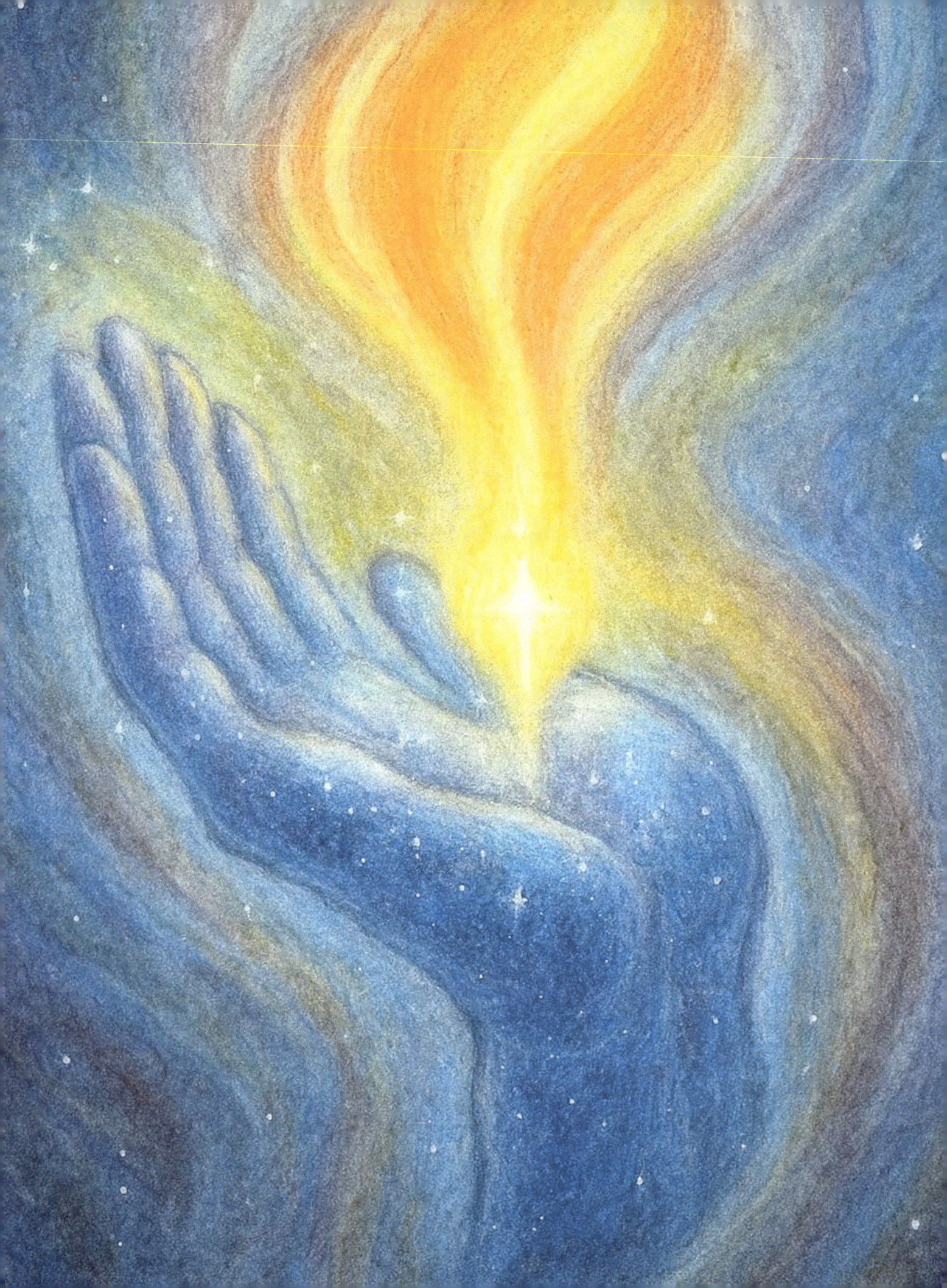

SELFLESS ACTION

Selfless action—or doing something purely for the sake of doing it as it is required by someone who cannot do it himself in given situation or time —generates genuine happiness. Here's why this works:

1. JOY WITHOUT EXPECTATION

When you volunteer or engage in any activity you love without expecting rewards, recognition, or outcomes, your mind is free from stress and comparison.
This freedom from attachment allows you to fully immerse in the activity, creating a natural sense of joy.

2. FLOW STATE

Engaging in something meaningful can put you in a flow state—a state of deep focus and presence. In flow, your mind stops wandering into worries or anxieties, and you experience pure contentment and satisfaction.

3. SENSE OF CONTRIBUTION

Even small acts of volunteering or helping others give you a sense of purpose.
Knowing your actions make a difference, however tiny, boosts self-worth and inner peace.

4. INNER TRANSFORMATION

Selfless acts cultivate empathy, compassion, and gratitude, qualities that naturally enhance happiness. Over time, this creates a habit of joy, independent of external circumstances.

5. UNIVERSAL PRINCIPLE

Many spiritual traditions—from the Vedas to modern psychology—emphasize that giving without expectation opens the heart and creates lasting happiness.
True contentment comes not from what you gain, but from the love, energy, and presence you share.

In short, volunteering or engaging in any selfless activity is like opening a door to inner joy and contentment—you give, yet you receive a far richer reward: peace of heart.

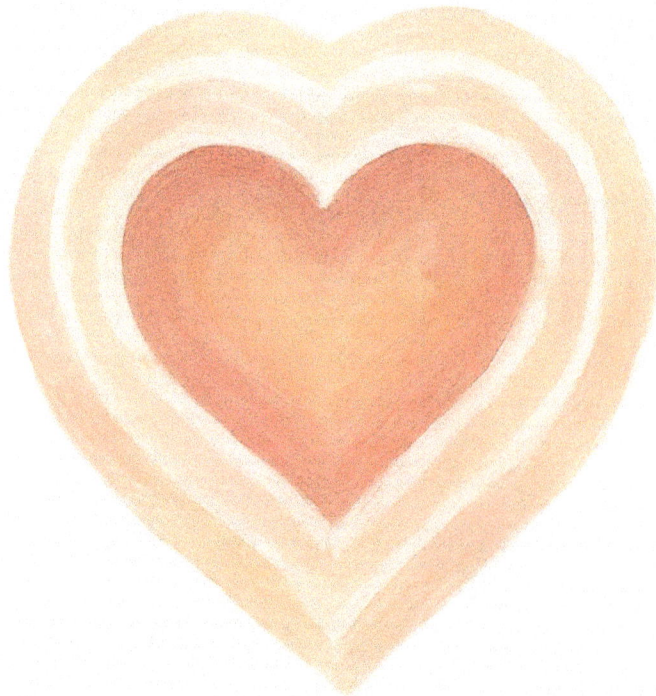

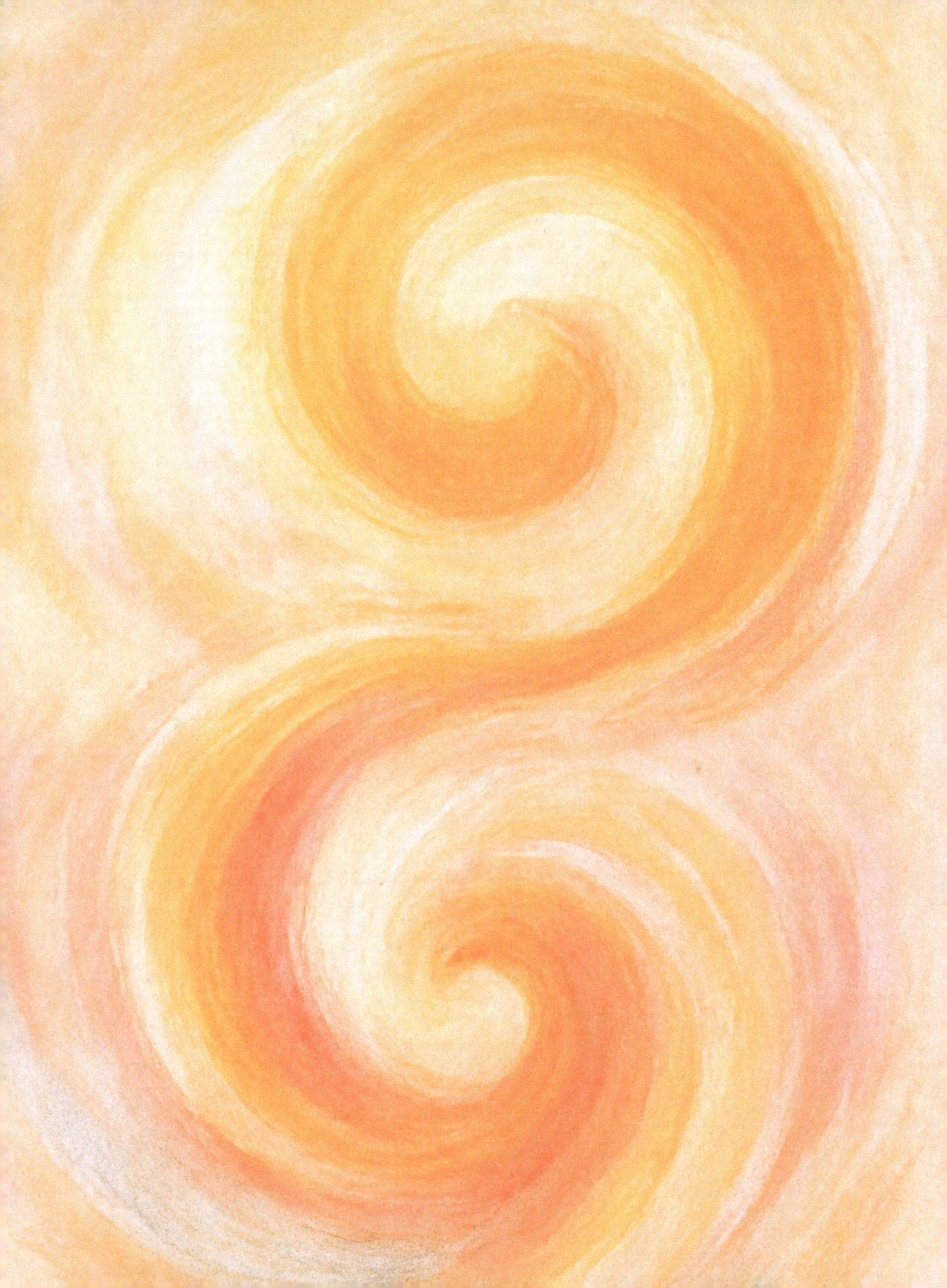

VOLUNTEERING

Volunteering in old age homes can also be deeply fulfilling, and there's a lot behind why it brings joy:

1. HUMAN CONNECTION

- Spending time with elderly people allows you to connect, listen, and share stories, creating meaningful relationships.
- Their wisdom and life experiences can be inspiring and grounding, giving you a fresh perspective on life.

2. EMOTIONAL FULFILLMENT

- Acts of kindness release endorphins and oxytocin, the "feel-good" chemicals in the brain, which naturally boost your mood.
- Simply seeing someone smile because of your presence can create a profound sense of satisfaction.

3. SENSE OF PURPOSE

- Volunteering provides a sense of meaning and contribution, reminding you that your actions have positive impact.
- Feeling needed and helpful contributes to inner peace and personal growth.

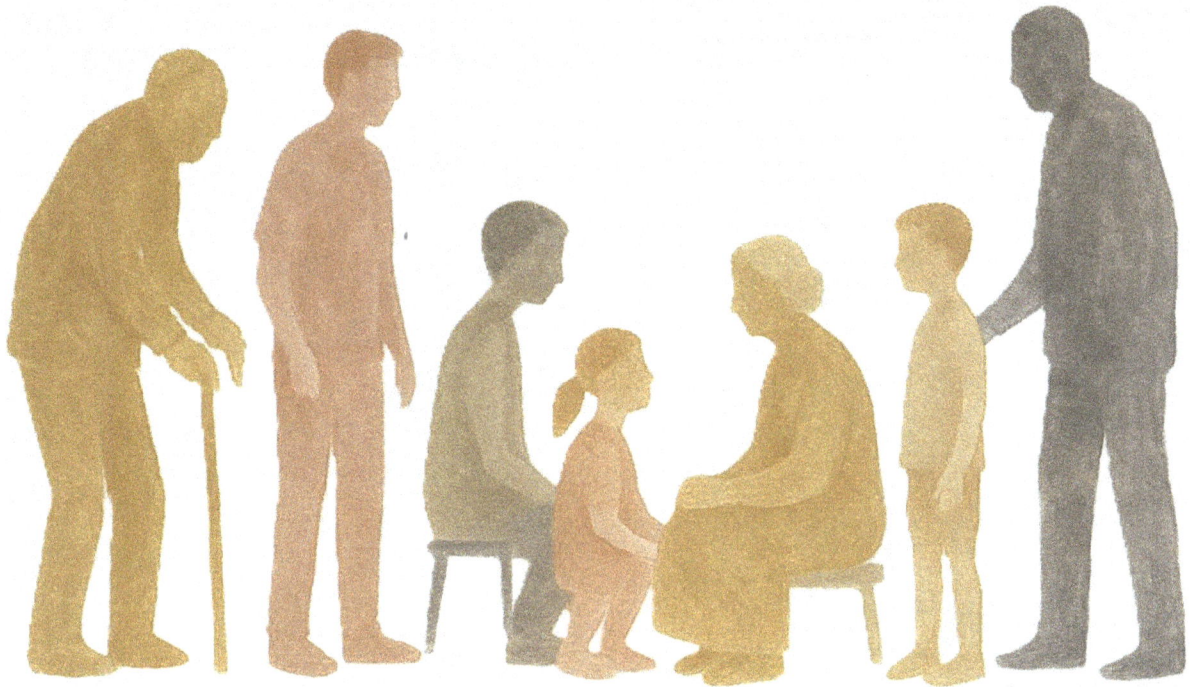

4. GRATITUDE AND PERSPECTIVE

- Spending time with elders can help you appreciate your own life circumstances and cultivate gratitude for small blessings.
- Their stories of resilience and life lessons can shift your mindset, making daily challenges feel more manageable.

5. MUTUAL JOY

- It's not just the elderly who benefit—volunteers often feel uplifted, energized, and emotionally enriched.
- Sharing laughter, music, games, or conversations creates a two-way exchange of joy.

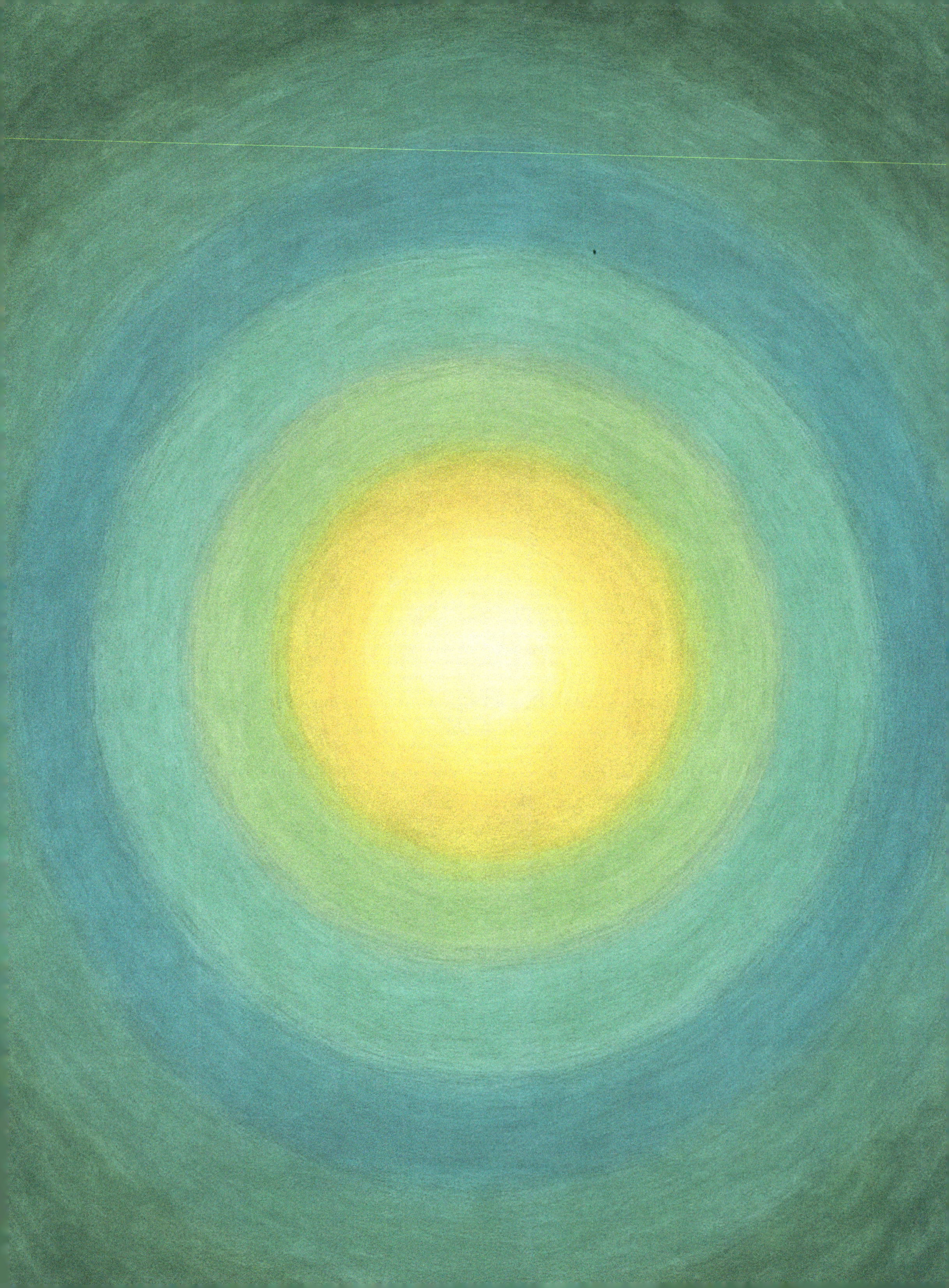

10 VEDIC STATEMENTS FOR BLISS

1. आनन्दो ब्रह्मेति व्यजानात् ।

"Ānando Brahmeti Vyajānāt" — He realized: Bliss is Brahman.

Story: The Potter and the Clay of Joy

Once, a humble potter asked a sage, "What is the source of this world?" The sage smiled and pointed to the clay in the potter's hands. "All your pots come from this one clay. The shapes differ, but the clay remains."

The potter nodded. "But what is the clay of the universe?"

The sage closed his eyes and said, "Ānanda — bliss. Just as your pots arise from clay, the universe arises from joy."

The potter began to see differently. Every sound of the wheel, every touch of the earth, every form he shaped was joy playing with itself. That night, as he rested, he felt — for the first time — that existence itself was smiling through him.

Moral: The universe is not born of struggle or duty, but of joy. When we rest in being, bliss reveals itself as the very ground of all creation.

2. सत्-चित्-आनन्द ।

"Sat–Chit–Ānanda" — Existence, Consciousness, Bliss — that is the Self.

Story: The Mirror and the Moon

A young monk spent years searching for enlightenment — he read scriptures, meditated in caves, and served the poor, yet peace eluded him. One night, he saw the full moon's reflection trembling in a pond.

He reached down to touch it, and the image scattered.

In that moment he realized — the moon was never in the water; it was always in the sky.

He laughed and wept at once. "So too," he said, "I am not the reflected form — this body, mind, or emotion — but the ever-present awareness that shines through them all."

Moral: You are not the reflection (your changing experiences), but the luminous sky of being that never ceases to shine — Sat (Being), Chit (Consciousness), and Ānanda (Bliss).

3. आनन्दं ब्रह्मणो विद्वान् न बिभेति कुतश्चन ।

"Ānandaṃ Brahmaṇo Vidvān Na Bibheti Kutaścana" — The knower of the bliss of Brahman fears nothing.

Story: The Lion Who Forgot Himself

A lion cub was raised among sheep. He bleated, grazed, and trembled at every sound.

One day, an old lion caught sight of him and dragged him to a still lake. "Look!" he said.

The cub saw his reflection beside the lion's — identical. A roar rose from within — deep, thunderous, liberating.

The sheep scattered in awe. From that day, the young lion never feared again, for he had seen what he truly was.

Moral: Fear vanishes not when the world changes, but when self-ignorance ends. The one who knows the Self as blissful Brahman moves through life fearless, free, and full of love.

4. आत्मानं विद्धि ।

"Ātmānam Vidhi" — Know Thyself.

Story: The Lost Necklace

A woman searched frantically for her pearl necklace — through her house, her garden, even the streets. Exhausted, she sat by a well. A friend approached and smiled, "Look at your neck."

There it was — the necklace she'd never lost.

Tears of relief flowed as she laughed, "All this while, I was searching for what I already am."

Moral: The Self is not to be found but recognized. When the search ends, what remains is truth — the simple joy of being yourself, infinite and whole.

5. यो वै भूम तत् सुखम् ।

"Yo Vai Bhūmā Tat Sukham" — The Infinite alone is bliss.

Story: The Surrender of the River

A young river flowed eagerly through valleys and plains, carrying its laughter and ripples along. One day, she reached the vast ocean and froze. "If I merge with that endless sea," she whispered, "will I lose who I am?" For a while, she held herself back, hugging the banks, afraid of losing her name, her journey, her identity. Yet the ocean's gentle waves called to her — not to take her away, but to welcome her into a greater whole.

Finally, with a trembling sigh, she let go. She merged with the ocean, feeling boundless, timeless peace. And yet, she noticed — she had not vanished. The ocean's water that rose as mist, became clouds, and then fell again as rain nourished her source, returning to the river's flow. Her identity remained, renewed by the very waters she had joined. Thus, she learned: surrender does not erase the self; it expands it. Joining the whole, she could still be herself — and her journey continued, endless, free, and infinite.

Moral: Finite pleasures fade because they are bound. Only when you dissolve your boundaries do you taste the bliss of the infinite.

6. आत्मना विन्दते वीर्यं, विद्यया विन्दते अमृतम् ।

"Ātmanā Vindate Vīryam, Vidyayā Vindate Amṛtam" — From the Self one gains strength; from wisdom, immortality.

Story: The Tree and the Wind

A young tree feared the fierce desert winds and tried to grow behind rocks for shelter. But it remained thin and weak. An old tree said, "Let the winds come. Face them — they will teach you strength."

The next storm bent the young tree almost to breaking. But its roots dug deeper, and its trunk grew firm. Years later, it stood unshaken, its branches singing in the same wind that once frightened it.

It realized: "My power came not from avoiding the storm, but from the Self that stood through it. My immortality is wisdom — knowing I am rooted beyond change."

Moral: True strength arises from inner stillness. Knowledge of the Self makes one fearless, free, and timeless.

7. आनन्दात् एव खल्विमानि भूतानि जायन्ते ।

"Ānandāt Eva Khalvimāni Bhūtāni Jāyante" — From bliss all beings are born, by bliss they live, into bliss they return.

Story: The River of Joy
A child once asked a sage, "Where do we come from?"

The sage took her to a river and said, "See how it flows from the mountains — that is birth. It dances through fields — that is life. It merges into the sea — that is return. The water is the same all along — only its forms change."

The child smiled. "So, life begins, flows, and ends in the same joy?"

"Yes," said the sage. "All beings are born from bliss, live by bliss, and return to bliss — just as the river never truly leaves the sea."

Moral: Existence is a circular dance of joy. When you remember your source, every movement becomes sacred.

8. आनन्दोऽहम् आनन्दोऽहम् ।

"Ānando'ham, Ānando'ham" — I am Bliss, I am Bliss itself.

Story: The Mask of Many Faces

A performer played many roles — king, beggar, warrior, saint — until one day he forgot who he was beneath the masks.

One night, before going on stage, he looked into the mirror and asked, "Who am I when the play ends?"

He removed one mask, then another, until none remained. What he saw was not a face, but light — vast, radiant, silent. A voice rose within: "Ānando'ham — I am bliss itself."

He went back to the stage, not as the actor lost in roles, but as the light behind them all.

Moral: Bliss is not an emotion; it is the recognition of your true identity beyond all roles and forms.

9. एष ह्येव आनंदयति ।

"Eṣa Hyev Ānandayati" — It is the Self alone that gives joy.

Story: The Music Box Reimagined

A woman inherited a delicate, antique music box from her grandmother. It was small and exquisitely carved, with tiny gears that clicked softly and a lid painted with golden flowers. Every evening, she would wind it carefully, letting its sweet, lilting tune fill her room.

At first, she delighted in it purely for its sound. Over time, however, she became attached — measuring her happiness by the music it produced. When the melody played, she felt joy; when it stopped, a shadow of emptiness followed.

One rainy evening, the music box refused to sing. She wound it again and again, but only silence emerged. Frustrated, she took it apart, examining the tiny gears and springs. But all she found were cold, silent metal parts. "Where is the music?" she asked the quiet room.

She sat back, exhausted and disappointed. And then, as the rain pattered softly on the windows, she noticed something subtle — a faint, warm vibration in her chest. At first she thought it was her heartbeat, but it was something more. It was steady, soft, and radiant — a deep, humming joy she had never paid attention to before.

Suddenly, she realized: the music had never truly come from the box. It had been a mirror, a channel through which her own inner harmony expressed itself. The melody had awakened a resonance already living within her — the Self itself, humming joy like a secret current in her heart.

She laughed, softly and freely, and felt tears of relief wash over her. The broken music box, instead of causing loss, had revealed a profound truth: happiness is not outside, waiting to be wound or earned; it is the Self, eternally playing its own song.

From that day forward, she still treasured the music box — now as a symbol, not the source. And whenever she felt anxious or restless, she would close her eyes and listen inward, hearing the familiar hum of her own joy.

Moral: The world's pleasures are mirrors. Joy is not something we chase; it is the music of our own Self, waiting to be recognized. When we stop seeking externally, the inner melody reveals itself — steady, radiant, and free from conditions.

10. आनन्दं ब्रह्म ।

"Ānandam Brahma" — Where there is no duality, there is bliss.

Story: The Wave and the Ocean

A little wave rose high on the sea, laughing as sunlight danced on her crest. But when she looked ahead, she saw waves crashing on the shore and grew terrified.

"Oh no," she cried, "we are all going to end!"

A deep, gentle voice rose from below — the Ocean itself.

"End? My dear one, you are not just a wave; you are me. You rise, you fall, you sparkle, but you never leave my being."

The wave grew still and felt the vastness beneath her — one endless expanse of water, moving as countless forms yet never divided. In that moment, she laughed again, not in excitement but in peace. "I am not the wave that comes and goes. I am the ocean that forever is."

Moral: When the sense of separation dissolves, fear and sorrow vanish. To know "I and the whole are one" is to taste the bliss that never fades — Ānandam Brahma.

ESSENCE OF THE TEN STATEMENTS

From bliss we are born,
by bliss we live,
in bliss we rest,
and bliss we ever are —
Sat–Chit–Ānanda.

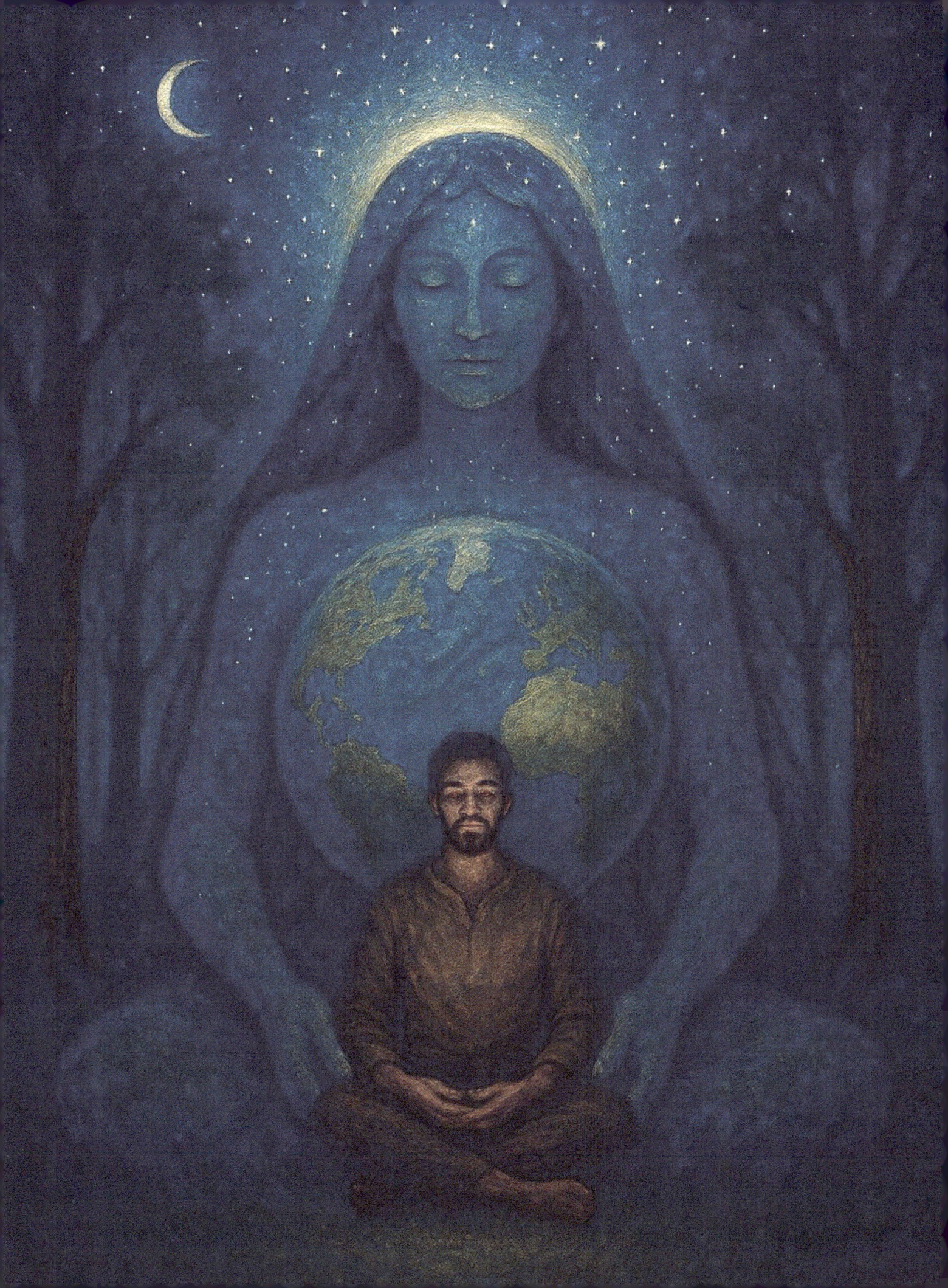

ABOUT THE AUTHOR

Rev. Dr. Gauri M Relan is an accomplished Holistic Healer, specializing in Natural, Vedic, and Metaphysical healing and has been healing since 1995 based on ancient Vedic philosophy of healing at Physical, Emotional, Mental and Spiritual level, so that there is total rejuvenation of physical health, emotional happiness with positive set of minds for one to finally grow spiritually. Dr. Gauri learnt various forms of Meditation and Energy healing techniques from Great Grand Masters of Reiki and Melchizedek and is a certified REIKI Master in Dr. Usui Mikao system.

Dr. Gauri did her Masters M.Sc (Botany), M.Phil (Wood Sciences & Forestry) from Himachal University Shimla, INDIA, 1992 and Ph.D from UMS, California, USA, plus numerous certification in Complimentary, Alternative & Integrative medicine from Harvard Medical School, Stanford and NIH- NCCAM (National Institutes of health - National Center for Complementary and Alternative Medicine) USA Gov. Dr Gauri was ordained as REVEREND by Wisdom of The Heart Church, California, USA, in the year 2010. She is a certified Yoga Instructor from SVYASA University, Bangalore, a certified NLP Master Practitioner & Numerologist from American university of NLP and Certified Hypnotist from American Alliance of Hypnotists.

Dr. Gauri is co-founder of Wellbeen Aeons Research Center Pvt. Ltd (www.wellbeen.com). She has authored many e-books on Apple iBooks and Amazon Kindle, APPS and many courses on UDEMY on Metaphysical self-help techniques. She has conducted numerous workshops in many corporate, many welfare clubs & societies, various schools and colleges in Bangalore. She conducts classes on YOGA, Reiki, Tarot and various Vedic and metaphysical methodologies.

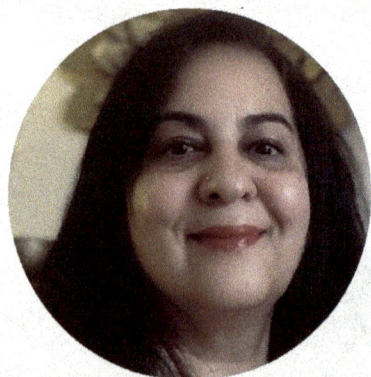

ABOUT THE DESIGNER

Sanyukta Shanbhag is a creative designer who transforms ideas into engaging visual experiences, blending layouts, color, and modern digital tools to make complex concepts feel intuitive and inviting.

Inspired by art, nature, and everyday details, she crafts visuals that spark curiosity, connect meaningfully with audiences, and leave a lasting impression.

❁ ❁ ❁ ❁ ❁

DISCLAIMER

The contents of this book are for informational purposes only and do not render any medical or psychological advice, opinion, diagnosis, or treatment. The information provided should not be used for diagnosing or treating a health problem or disease and no attempt is being made to provide diagnosis, care, treatment, or rehabilitation of individuals, or apply medical, mental health or human development principles to provide diagnosing, treating, operating, or prescribing for any human disease, pain, injury, deformity, or physical condition.

The statements and the products have not been evaluated by FDA and the services and products are not intended to diagnose, treat, cure or prevent any disease or medical condition. The information contained herein is not intended to replace a one-on-one relationship with a doctor or qualified health professional. Any techniques address only the underlying spiritual issues to address energetic blockages that may have an impact on wellness and energetic balance, facilitating the body's natural ability to bring itself to homeostasis, which may have an impact on health and well-being. This book is not a substitute for professional health care. If you have or suspect you may have a medical or psychological problem, you should consult your appropriate health care provider. Never disregard professional medical advice or delay in seeking it because of something you have read on this website. Links on this website are provided only as an informational resource, and it should not be implied that we recommend, endorse or approve of any of the content at the linked sites, nor are we responsible for their availability, accuracy or content. Any review or other matter that could be regarded as a testimonial or endorsement does not constitute a guarantee, warranty, or prediction regarding the outcome of any consultation. The testimonials on this website represent the anecdotal experience of individual consumers. Individual experiences are not a substitute for scientific research.